Polycystic Ovary Syndrome: Fighting Back !

A Lifestyle Manual

2nd Edition

Angela Kay Dotson

Sparhawk Health Publications
Boston

Sparhawk Health Publications   Boston

Dotson, Angela Kay.
  Polycystic Ovary Syndrome: Fighting Back! 2nd Edition

  1. Woman's Health
I. Title.
ISBN 0-9705025-1-6

**For Michael,
Who kept the wind in my sails and
gave me a port in stormy weather**

TABLE OF CONTENTS

**When you come to the end of your rope,
tie a knot and hang on.**

*Franklin D. Roosevelt
1882-1945, Thirty-second President of the USA*

Chapter 1
In the Beginning

Much has happened since the first edition of this book - both in the world of Polycystic Ovary Syndrome (PCOS) and also in my own life. More doctors, although sadly not all, are recognizing that aggressive treatment of PCOS is a good thing. Still, there seems to be a disparity from doctor to doctor about the best approach. I've gone from being single to getting married and trying to conceive. Perhaps more than ever I am really facing the syndrome. At this writing, I have been trying to conceive for seven months. I am taking metformin (glucaphage) and hoping for the best. Even though the first edition has been unavailable for several months, I still get e-mails begging for information.

The purpose of this book, as was the first edition, remains to educate those suffering with PCOS, the public, and potential PCOS patients who have yet to be diagnosed with the condition. I also hope that physicians, spouses, and other family members will read this book in order to better understand the unique challenges that women with PCOS (and teenagers as well) encounter on a daily basis.

One of my earliest memories as a fourth grader was trying to hide the large whitehead that formed in the middle of the night on the tip of my nose. My older brother of two years kindly pointed it out by shrieking and yelling something appropriate like "Oh, gross! I'm going to tell Mom." I responded by enclosing myself in the bathroom and squeezing until the ugly thing popped. If I hadn't accomplished the feat, my mother would have.

On a nightly basis, she picked, pinched, squeezed and poked my bumps in an effort to rid my young face of them. Afterwards she dabbed on over-the-counter acne products, medications that failed to diminish the spots that caused my classmates to wonder why my "chicken pox" hadn't gone away. Unfortunately, I suffered in spite of the face washings, squeezings and medications.

In addition, I became aware that my budding breasts strained at my thin shirts and caused the boys to stare. The training bra, when duly installed by my mother, seemed to cause as much attention as the breasts. Irony prevailed in my teenage years when I realized that I would never develop beyond small breasts, much to my great consternation.

Instead of giving me voluptuous breasts, my body chose to give me lots and lots of hair. My mother let me start shaving when I was about ten years old and I found that I needed to shave my legs and arm pits on a daily basis because the hair grew so thickly. To my embarrassment, hair also grew around my nipples and in a line from my navel to my pubic area. By the time I was fourteen I was bleaching and tweezing on a regular basis.

At age nine, strange fleeting abdominal pains caused me to double over. My mother's reaction was to send me in a hurry to the bathroom where I was instructed to check my panties. At the time I had no idea what exactly I was checking for. I had read the book for young girls my mother gave me; however, the principles of menstruation in the book and checking my panties did not really click until two years later when I actually saw blood for the first time. Several months after my eleventh birthday, the event finally arrived. I experienced sharp pains at the dinner table and rushed to the bathroom where I stared in disbelief at the bright red stains on my panties. Panicked and proud at the same time, I yelled for my mother until she came running into the bathroom. The second phase had started. Little did I know that day what I was in for.

That first period lasted an incredible three weeks. During that time I bled heavily and the cramping was often nearly unbearable. Some days I had trouble getting out of bed. My mother, thinking that I was exaggerating my symptoms, told me that I needed to learn to deal with this.   Didn't all women suffer?   Of course, my mother had endometriosis so her own irregular bleeding and pain probably made mine seem normal. After awhile, I conditioned myself to expect periods that lasted a minimum of ten to fourteen days for the first couple of years.

My weight became an issue as I thickened, especially my belly and waist, causing relatives to comment on my "stockiness". In spite of everything I tried to do, I seemed to pack on the pounds, gaining an amazing twenty pounds in the seventh grade alone. I exercised as much as two hours straight every night, doing hundreds of sit ups and leg lifts. In the summer, I ate tiny portions and spent hours bicycling up and down the dirt roads around our house. Yet the weight wouldn't budge.

Almost two years later, during the summer when I was thirteen, I bled continuously for two months straight. At first I hid the fact from my mother. By the time I blurted out that I had been bleeding for that long, she almost didn't believe me. However, I wound up in a doctor's office shortly thereafter for my first pelvic exam. The doctor was extremely kind and gentle. He apologized for the necessity of giving me a pelvic exam at such an early age. He had no choice. I was surrounded by kind and sympathetic nurses who wrapped my feet warmly in the stirrups and made sure that I was comfortable as possible. While he examined me, the doctor spoke to me, engaging me in conversation about my schoolwork so that I didn't focus entirely on his actions. When he finished, and I had dressed, he told my mother and I his suspicion that I was not ovulating. I was too young, however, for him to be sure. He prescribed birth control pills for a limited time to get my body on track. He hoped that the pills would jumpstart my hormones into working properly.

When I was later taken off the pill, however, the problems returned. I was now under the care of another physician (the former having moved away) and he constantly reassured me that I would "outgrow" all my problems. The lengthy and painful periods returned. The spring that I turned fifteen, the doctor took drastic measures when pills failed to get the bleeding to stop. I had my first "D and C" (dilatation and curettage).

The doctor explained that he would perform an out-patient surgery in which he would give me a local anesthetic before dilating my cervix so that he could access and scrape the lining of my uterus to remove any tissues to stop the bleeding. Apprehensive, I found myself having the procedure minutes later. I awakened to excruciating pain some time later and realized that the anesthetic had worn off before the doctor had completed the procedure. With a nurse helping to restrain me while he finished, the doctor profusely offered his apologies. The extent of the scar tissue that he was removing was far greater than he had anticipated.

I endured the rest of the procedure and then was sent home to rest for a few days. Then I went back on the pill again and the pain and duration of my periods began to subside. In fact, by the time I was a senior in high school, I had stopped having periods altogether except for some slight spotting occasional. And incredibly, though I never connected the events until much later, my weight began slowly coming off in response to diet and exercise.

I was not alarmed by the infrequency or absence of a period at the time. Indeed, after the painful long periods from before I was thrilled to be free from them. It was not until my second year of college that I began to take the matter more seriously. I had not had a period in over six months. In fact, on average, I had ceased having more than one period per year. A close friend, telling me that an absolute absence of menstruation was surely some sign of a problem, encouraged me to seek out a doctor's advice.

I was referred by the college doctor to a physician in town. At first he seemed puzzled. He asked me what I thought were very strange questions. Did I shave frequently? When had I started my period? What were my first periods like? Finally, he told me that he thought he knew what was wrong with me and asked me to get dressed. This was in 1987 and I was twenty years old. The doctor informed me that he thought I had what was referred to as Stein-Leventhol Syndrome (now known as Polycystic Ovary Syndrome). My diagnosis was difficult, he said, because I was not overweight. What aroused his suspicion was that one of my ovaries felt enlarged and swollen. He had recently treated another patient with the similar condition. I did not tell him that I was barely eating in order to keep my weight down and that I exercised frequently.

He suggested viewing my ovaries via laparoscopy in order to make a definitive diagnosis. If he found tiny cysts covering the ovaries he would perform a "pie wedge reduction", a procedure used at that time to help treat the condition. Almost by accident, researchers had discovered that removing a small section of the ovary for inspection at the lab often seemed to alleviate some of the symptoms. A few weeks later, I arrived at the hospital where blood was drawn and where I was prepped for surgery. The surgery was a blur and I was in and out of consciousness until the next evening. When I awoke at last I was told that I had Stein-Leventhol Syndrome.

I expected some sort of miracle from the surgery but was clearly misguided. The first period came, as predicted, on a normal schedule and lasted for a normal duration. After that, however, my periods became erratic and extremely painful. The cramping at times was so severe that I tried ridiculous positions to try to alleviate the pain - sometimes hanging with my head dangling over the bed with my legs stretched straight up in the air, in hopes that some sort odd positioning would end my agony.

During this same time, I also began the battle with my weight again, gaining close to twenty pounds that year alone. I lost my self -esteem and struggled with feelings of self-loathing and depression, never associating my condition with my weight difficulties. At the time, my doctor had said that Stein-Leventhol Syndrome (again, this was the former name for Polycystic Ovary Syndrome) was a fertility issue and that I should have no other concerns about my overall health because the condition did not pose any other health risks. I continued to believe this explanation over the next eleven years until, by chance, I happened to see an article in "Good Housekeeping" magazine in November 1998.

Stunned, I learned that not only was PCOS related to an over-production of insulin, but that I was at risk for diabetes, heart disease and endometrial cancer. First, I experienced fear. No one had ever told me that my condition could potentially prove to be such a serious health threat. It seemed quite unfair that on top of my infertility I was being hit with increased risks of diabetes, heart disease and endometrial cancer.

Secondly, I was excited to learn that there might be a way out. If insulin was the problem, I would just ask my doctor to prescribe the diabetic medications I read about that were being tested. Then the second blow came. Even though many doctors believe that the condition can be helped by these drugs, the Food and Drug Administration had not yet approved them for use by women with PCOS. There were also concerns about the safety of these drugs.

What could I do? I began looking for clinical research studies. The first one that I contacted informed me that I was a good candidate except that I lacked one qualification; I was not obese by clinical standards. Disappointed, I contacted another study, hoping that any information obtained by such a study would improve my chances of better treatment. I began a study at Brigham and Women's Hospital in Boston after first abstaining from the birth control pill for three months. The researchers wanted to see what was going on when I was completely off of hormones.

In hindsight, it was a terrible decision for me. My weight immediately increased and I began to feel tired, cranky and irritable. I stayed bloated and experienced feelings of despair and anxiety. At the beginning of the fourth month I went in for my first battery of tests. The results included the following elevated levels of testosterone and triglycerides:

total testosterone: 116 ng/dl
(normal levels are 20-58 ng/dl)

free testosterone: 44 ng/dl
(normal levels are 1-15 ng/dl)

triglycerides: 393 mg/dl
(normal levels are 35-135 mg/dl)

In addition to that, I had begun bleeding. This bleeding continued for three months and resulted in another D&C, after which my regular physician advised that I drop out of the study. Her exam reinforced the finding of elevated testosterone levels, as well as a complete cessation of estrogen production. She ordered an immediate prescription of hormone treatment and I chose the birth control pill because my body was used to it, or so I thought. The next month proved difficult; I experienced cramping, nausea, fatigue, mood swings resulting in crying for no reason, and constant bloating. Fortunately, I weathered the month and began to feel more positive effects the following month.

Fast forward to today. Metformin (glucaphage) is now available as an off-label drug by some physicians. I take glucaphage daily and will continue to do so until I, hopefully, get pregnant. After pregnancy I plan to resume the glucaphage again since I have experienced positive results with it including more normal hormones, normal periods and fewer attacks of low blood sugar. I still continue having problems with high cholesterol and high triglycerides but am trying to manage those with diet and exercise.

One of the frustrations I experienced upon my initial diagnosis was a lack of information about the condition of PCOS. I combed through libraries and bookstores when I was first diagnosed and could never find any books written to the patient of this condition. I later learned that this was because none existed. As I talked to others who also suffered from this condition, it became obvious that there was a need for such a book. While there are now other books available, this lifestyle manual attempts to help women understand what PCOS is, what can be done to alleviate the effects of the condition, and how to gain control of at least how one reacts to the condition. I have included everything that I always wanted to know but could not find in any bookstore.

I emphasize that I am not a doctor and do not advocate using this manual in lieu of any physician's advice. Rather, I hope that this manual will help identify new sufferers of PCOS and serve as a supplemental form of information for those who have already been diagnosed with PCOS. Consult your physician for questions on dietary concerns or before starting any exercise program.

**When life knocks you down, try to land on your back.
Because if you can look up, you can get up.
Let your reason get you back up.**

Les Brown
1945-, American Speaker, Author, Trainer, Motivator Lecturer

Chapter 2
It's Not Your Fault!

If you are like me, all your life you have been scolded about your weight gains and figure flaws. When you tried to explain that you really *did* stick to your diet, did anyone believe you? When you exercised for just as long as your best friend, only to lose little or no weight, did you get the feeling that no one believed you? Did you stop exercising because you thought "what's the point?" Did you hopelessly try to explain that those fifteen pounds just *appeared* in spite of the fact that your eating habits had not changed? If you answered yes to any of these questions then you are not alone! Prepare for a surprise. It's not your fault!

Now wait. Don't get too excited. People will *still* think that you are coming up with excuses even if you tell them that Polycystic Ovary Syndrome causes your weight problems. Be prepared to hear that you just haven't tried hard enough. Or they may agree that your condition *caused* your weight problems but that traditional methods of weight loss will still work. Forget about trying to convince them otherwise. Instead, ignore fad diets and miracle pills, which don't work in the long run. Prepare yourself to wage one of the toughest battles of your life. This battle, incidentally, is not merely one for cosmetic purposes. Patients with PCOS also face dramatic health issues including heart disease, diabetes and endometrial cancer. We are fighting for our very lives. Being slender and athletic is just a nice side effect of healthier bodies. The reality is that PCOS makes you susceptible to obesity due to the body's inability to absorb sugar properly. Note that I am being very simplistic here; in later chapters I will detail more of the problems your body encounters, especially in light of the over-production of insulin.

For the moment, you should concentrate on letting go all of the guilt you've built up for not being able to lose weight. Take a deep breath and hold it for a few seconds. Now let it out and feel your body relaxing. Close your eyes and allow yourself one final look at those negative thoughts and feelings that you've harbored against your body. You know what I'm talking about. All those nasty looks you gave your body when you glanced in a mirror. Admit it. Haven't you harbored a few thoughts of self-loathing and disgust? I know I have at several points in my life. Looking in the mirror I would generate a substantial amount of self-pity and sadness that my body did not conform to the slender image I wanted it to.

I am no longer unkind to the image in the mirror. Although I still face day to day challenges of PCOS, I have changed my attitude of self-defeat. PCOS is a challenge, not a sentence. Instead of working against my body, seeing the image in the mirror as my mortal enemy, I now see a part of myself that wants just as much to get in shape as my mind wants it to. My body likes being able to run up the stairs without being winded; it delights in letting go of stress and relaxing into a deep soothing slumber at night; it thrills at moving with energy and confidence.

At one point a few years ago, my body was at it's worst level. I had stopped taking the birth control pill to be in a PCOS study conducted by Brigham and Women's University in Boston. I gained fifteen pounds in one month. I craved sugar to the extent that an hour after I ate I wanted to eat again. My appetite knew no bounds. I was sluggish, irritable, overweight and depressed. My testosterone levels had risen sharply and my estrogen production had ceased. I bled for several weeks, although the amount was small. Feeling as though my body had gone completely out of control, I sought the advice of my physician who recommended that I drop out of the study. (Please note that studies like these are important to helping PCOS patients. Individual experiences may differ from my own.)

Fortunately, my health began to improve after I resumed taking the birth control pill. I could feel the difference after about a month as my hormone levels were forced back into sync. After that experience, however, I got angry. I decided that I would not let this condition determine my state of mind. In addition, I would fight to gain control over the condition of my body.

A new problem cropped up later, however, as I suddenly became besieged by debilitating migraines. When I casually mentioned them to my physician (a new one under a new health provider) she became alarmed and requested that I stop taking the pill immediately. When I told her what had happened the last time I stopped taking them she agreed to speak to an endocrinologist about my request to take glucaphage instead since I had heard that it could regulate periods. Imagine my surprise when the endocrinologist - who had never personally even met me - refused. He said that he would only allow me to go on the drug if I was trying to get pregnant. My doctor called me back and said that I would have to rethink the situation and perhaps go back on the birth control pill. I was flabergasted! This was the doctor who had told me that the birth control pill was unsafe for continued use because of the migraines. Incidentally, this particular physician had not even heard of PCOS. When I explained the condition to her she noted that it was "interesting."

At this point I got angry. I demanded a second opinion. I gave her the name of an endocrinologist I had heard about and insisted that she gain me a referral. I got the referral and was rewarded with an endocrinologist who knew all about pcos. She was more than happy to prescribe the glucaphage to me. I went home happy and then was socked with a letter from my insurance provider saying that they had agreed to the one consultation but that my physician should take over my continued treatment from there on. Once again I was angry. My primary care physician knew nothing about either pcos or the drug that I was taking. How was she going to treat me effectively? Fortunately, it was during a time of year when I could change my insurance provider and I hastily did so. My new physician was very competent and referred me promptly to an endocrinologist even though she was also available to see me. I include this just so that you are motivated to fight for your rights as a patient if you need to do so. If your physician is not knowledgeable about pcos or is unwilling or able to refer you to an endocrinologist find someone else. My doctor was nice but "nice" wasn't going to make me healthy.

While you are trying to ensure your health via struggling for proper medical treatment, however, make sure that you do not wage war against yourself. Your body is doing the best it can and needs special treatment. You must consider and treat your body as a special vessel. Imagine if you put rocks or marbles in your favorite blender. The results would be disastrous. If the blender didn't short out you can be sure that the insides of it would be damaged, if not destroyed. Our bodies react much the same way when we pour ingredients into them that they are not capable of processing. Keep in mind that your body can not handle foods the way that a normal person can. You may match the eating and exercise patterns of a slender, healthy person. Yet, while she loses weight, you gain several pounds.

We could blame the world or ourselves that we don't have a "model" that is sufficient for handling some of the same ingredients that other "models" seem to accept. And in a way, that is exactly what I used to do. I spent a lot of energy deploring the fact that my body couldn't keep off excess weight eating the same things as other people ate. The problem is that blaming or feeling self-pity or pointing a finger at our medical condition doesn't change a thing. Until a magic pill is invented, women with PCOS are going to continue to struggle with weight and other health issues.

So let's accept that fact. And *move on!* You'll notice I speak a lot about motivation. The reason is that you will need to get yourself motivated on a daily basis for an indefinite amount of time. If you are looking for a quick fix, then this book is not for you. Changing eating and exercise habits takes time to develop. This book is not about superficial diets or exercise programs that you follow for a few weeks and then stop. Rather, this book is a life changing system that requires developing diet and exercise patterns to best suit the special needs of patients with Polycystic Ovary Syndrome. Incidentally, if you are taking medications, including glucaphage, exercise and diet are still important. As always, though, consult your doctor before pursuing any exercise or diet program. Now let's jump right into exploring our attitudes and its effect on our health.

**Nothing has any power over me other than
that which I give it through my conscious thoughts.**

Anthony Robbins
1960-, American Author, Speaker,
Peak Performance Expert / Consultant

Chapter 3
Mental Attitude

You may be wondering why I've included a chapter on mental attitude. After all, your attitude didn't make you sick in the first place. Yet, attitude will determine whether you control your illness or whether your illness controls you. Researchers have long suspected that mental attitude plays a great role in whether or not a person stays healthy. For example, research indicates that seniors who live the longest tend to be those persons who have positive attitudes toward life and who stay active. Because mood swings are often an inevitable part of the life of PCOS sufferers, staying upbeat and positive is essential.

Anthony Robbins, a motivational speaker, teaches in his *Personal Power* motivational tape series that our moods can be altered if we learn to "use state changes." [46] What typically happens is that we learn to associate certain people, actions, etc. with how we feel. For example, if I am sad, I may start recalling sad things that have happened in my life. Such thoughts may prompt memories of past failures. Soon I may become so sad that I will cry for an hour.

Could I stop that? Yes. By using state changes I would change my physiology to stop the sad mood before it progressed beyond control. What could I do? As soon as I felt sad I could change my posture, raise my head, laugh, go for a walk, rent a funny movie or call a good friend (one who won't let me gripe and complain the whole time). It is easy to feel sorry for yourself when you have any sort of illness.

Being told that PCOS is a lifelong condition is not a cheery prospect. However, it is not the end of the world. PCOS is controllable. We can live normal, productive lives. Happiness is achieved by focusing on the positive aspects of your life rather than the negative ones. Having PCOS will help you to be more empathetic to others with lifelong illnesses. In addition, you have the opportunity to affect the quality of life imposed by this condition. Make the challenge of having PCOS the catalyst to make your life better and healthier.

I know what you're thinking. *Better? Healthier?* No, I'm not insane. I can honestly say that at the present time I am eating healthier than I ever have before. That doesn't mean that I don't have bouts of the munchies or that I don't pig out sometimes on dessert. But I no longer eat an entire package of oreo cookies either or a quarter pound of m&m's in one day (something I have to confess that I use to do quite often). My energy levels have improved and I rarely suffer from low blood sugar attacks (hypoglycemia). I no longer feel compelled to raid the refrigerator an hour after dinner. I exercise more regularly and like my body more than ever before. Is my body perfect? No. I'd still like to lose that elusive 10 pounds. But I am also in the range of healthy weight for my age and height. Most importantly, though, I no longer feel like a victim!

Before eliminating large amounts of sugar from my diet, I often felt like a slave chained to food. The quick bouts of pleasure I experienced from sugar highs (ice cream, candy, cookies, etc.) were always followed by feelings of guilt and anxiety. I felt guilty because I couldn't control my eating and anxious because I worried about gaining additional weight.

I do have some tricks up my sleeve, though. I discovered Splenda®, a sugar substitute, that has no calories and works just like sugar. That means that I can make myself hot chocolate and not feel one bit of guilt. I can also drink kool-aide again. When I want chocolate I make sure it is worth the eating. I like really dark chocolate so I try to only indulge when I can get the good stuff (or make it). I use "heart healthy" margarine and I use low-sugar products when I can find them. I haven't stopped eating. Instead I've tried to make as many healthier substitutions as I can. I know that I will always like ice cream so I get the "no sugar added" variety when I can't help myself. Let's be realistic. Most of us are never going to be able to give up sweets entirely. If you can, I say great for you! The rest of us have to learn moderation and substitution.

Exercise also helped me to feel stronger and more powerful. Conquering physical obstacles helps me to know that I can conquer other battles in life. For example, just a couple of years ago I was unable to do a single regular pushup. I always told myself that women were not built for pushups, that many of my friends probably couldn't do them either. Still, I always felt weak in my upper body. In the back of my mind, I faulted myself that I was not capable of such a task. Even though I was exercising, I never ventured past the bent-knee push up. On one level doing a full pushup is not really a big deal. In my case, however, the push up represented a physical obstacle that my mind had convinced me that I could never perform.

At some point along the way, I *gave up trying*. Until I stopped trying, my many unsuccessful attempts at push ups were not failures. They only became failures when I no longer tried to succeed. That all changed one day as I read a woman's magazine that encouraged those of us who performed bent knee pushups to venture into a full body pushup. On a whim, without a lot of enthusiasm, I got on the floor and prepared myself to fail once again. I had only allowed myself a glimmer of hope that I could perhaps do a partial one. Imagine my surprise and elation when my body responded to the challenge and, though probably not with the best form, managed not one pushup but three!

That moment, as ridiculous as it might sound, was one of the greatest moments in my life. I had turned an impossible task into an achievable act. Whatever your "impossible" thing to do is, try to tackle it bit by bit. Maybe you've always wanted to learn to swim but were afraid. Or maybe walking around the block would be enough to give you a heart attack but you'd love to do a three-mile charity walk. Break up the ultimate goal into smaller tasks and just try. Sign up for a swimming lesson at the local YMCA. Make a chart and walk half a block this week and add 100 steps every day. My challenge to you is to find your weakness and turn it into one of your most powerful assets. Once you take an impossible task and make yourself overcome obstacles to succeed, you will always have confidence in yourself and your abilities.

I don't hate my body any longer because my body should not be punished if I put bad things into it or neglect it by forcing it to sit slumped on the living room sofa while I watch endless hours of television. What I did with that anger was to use it to motivate myself. My current enemies are inactivity and lack of attention to diet. Make them your enemies as well. Get mad. Take action and take control!

Prepare yourself to wage a constant battle. The less you exercise, the easier inactivity can lure you with such devious methods as procrastination, excuses, and other activities. If the thought of cleaning your bathroom suddenly seems more important than exercising, be vigilant. Remember that you are fighting for your life!

When you are tempted to not exercise or to ignore proper diet, remember what lies ahead: increased risks for obesity, heart disease and diabetes. Exercise is thought to decrease one's chances of developing these conditions by keeping weight to acceptable levels.

You've probably heard that "eating sugar makes you want sugar." There is a great deal of truth in this simple statement. Keep this in mind when you are tempted by that donut or candy bar. You won't be satisfied with just one. In fact, your body will mercilessly cry out for more, even against your best will power. Realize that sugar is a poison for your body and avoid it. Fortunately, the food industry has begun to provide some tempting alternatives. However, if you find yourself overeating no matter what you eat, that issue needs to be addressed as well. Make sure that you are not eating out of boredom or emotional distress. Later in the book I'll go over how keeping a journal can help you see why you eat as well as what you eat.

Ready to move on? Let's start out by exploring Polycystic Ovary Syndrome. Once you understand how the condition disrupts your health, then we can focus on how to fight back for control of our bodies.

If we could give every individual the right amount of
nourishment and exercise, not too little and not too much,
we would have found the safest way to health.

Hippocrates
Ancient Greek Physician

Chapter 4
What is Polycystic Ovarian Syndrome?

A definition.

Polycystic Ovary Syndrome, a condition marked by multiple cysts building up inside the ovaries, is a hormonal disorder associated with infertility, acne, excess hair growth, amenhorrea (absence of menstruation), weight gain (especially around the middle of the torso - known as "apple shaped") and an overproduction of insulin which can lead to other serious conditions such as insulin-resistance, diabetes, heart disease and endometrial cancer[1].

How common is the condition?

Between 5 and 10 percent of women in the United States are affected with PCOS and the disorder is "probably the most common hormonal abnormality in women of reproductive age."[2] However, this number may be an under representation of the women who actually have PCOS. Not all women with PCOS have the same exact symptoms (or even every single symptom) and many women remain undiagnosed. Because the figures of current percentages of women with PCOS are mostly derived from reproductive clinics, many women who have not been diagnosed due to never seeking fertility treatments, will not be included.[3]

In England and Austria, where population-based studies have been conducted, the percentage of those affected by PCOS has been estimated at 20-25%. [4]

Why have I not heard of this condition before?

The disorder can be difficult to diagnose, as in my case, because the symptoms are often attributed to other conditions. Dr. Andrea Dunaif, MD, Chief of the Division of Women's Health at Boston's Brigham and Women's Hospital writes: "For many years, many physicians have dismissed PCOS as a cosmetic problem, or one that interfered 'only' with a woman's ability to get pregnant. We now know that PCOS affects far more than reproduction." [5]

Why should I be concerned?

"Polycystic Ovary Syndrome sufferers experience greater risks of developing coronary disease, diabetes and endometrial cancer." [6]

- **Heart Disease**

  The incidence of high insulin levels (like those associated with women with PCOS) is often associated with risk factors known to contribute to heart attack or stroke: low levels of good cholesterol (HDL); high levels of other fat-carrying molecules known as triglycerides; and high blood pressure. [7]

  The risk of myocardial infarction and ischaemic heart disease is seven times that of other women. [8]

- **Diabetes**

  Discussing her research at Brigham and Women's Hospital in Boston, Dr. Dunaif writes: "My colleagues and I have found that up to 30 percent of women with PCOS have impaired glucose-tolerance, a major risk factor for type 2 (adult-onset) diabetes and heart disease; 7.5 percent of women under age 45 with PCOS actually have type 2 diabetes compared with 1 percent of women this age without PCOS." [9]

- **Endometrial Cancer**

High androgen levels in women with PCOS prevent the regular, natural shedding of the lining of the uterus (the endometrium) each month, leading to the risk of the development of endometrial cancer early in life. [10]

What are some of the symptoms of PCOS?

Symptoms of PCOS can vary greatly but may include hirsutism (excessive hair growth on the face, chest, abdomen, etc.), hair loss (androgenic alopecia, in a classic "male baldness" pattern); acne; polycystic ovaries; obesity; infertility or reduced fertility.[11] Central obesity ("apple-shape") is typical with women with PCOS. [12] "83 percent of women who have severe acne also have PCOS." [13]

Other symptoms are insulin resistance, insulin secretory defects, and glucose intolerance.[14] Insulin resistance, as will be covered in more detail later in the book, is thought to be the cause of PCOS and is linked to other ill effects.[15]

When do the symptoms of PCOS appear?

While some women do not develop symptoms until their early to mid-20's, symptoms frequently appear in adolescence, around the start of menstruation. [16]

How do you get PCOS?

Many researchers are studying the effects of genetics in the role of the development of PCOS. Several genes are thought to be involved. [17] IRS and INS, genes that regulate the insulin receptor and insulin expression; the OB (obesity) gene; and the HLA Dqal (glycogen synthetase) gene are currently being studied.[18] In addition, CYP17 and CYP19 (enzymes regulating androgen production and action), are also being studied. [19]

Another interesting theory was postulated by researchers in the United Kingdom. They presented their findings in The Lancet, on October 17, 1997, about their study in which the prevalence of polycystic ovaries and the plasma concentrations of gonadotropin hor-mones and androgens were related to the women's body size at birth and the length of gestation. [20] Two hundred thirty-five (235) women aged 40 to 42 years were studied and 49 (21 percent) of the women had polycystic ovaries.[21] The study indicated that obese, hirsute women with PCOS have higher than normal ovarian secretion of androgens that is associated with high birth weight and maternal obesity while thin women with PCOS have altered control of LH release resulting from prolonged gestation.[22] The research, though not yet duplicated, could lead to a greater understanding of PCOS and its cause.[23]

How is PCOS diagnosed?

Doctors frequently have difficulty diagnosing PCOS because there is no single, quick test to identify the syndrome. [24]

Some of the diagnostic tools used, as compiled by the University of Chicago, are as follows:

- "A detailed patient history.

- Ultrasound to check for enlarged or cystic ovaries.

- Blood tests, to detect elevated levels of androgens.

- Blood test to detect high levels of LH (luteinizing hormone) or an elevation in the ratio of LH to FSH (follicle stimulating hormone).

- Monitoring of the ovary's response to either a stimulatory dose of gonadotropin-releasing hormone agonist or a suppressive dose of medications such as dexamethasone.

- The physician will also try to rule out other possible causes of irregular menstruation and excessive hair growth, such as Cushing's syndrome, congenital adrenal hyperplasia, or other disorders of the pituitary or adrenal glands." [25]

How is PCOS treated?

The symptoms that a woman complains of when seeking medical advice are the ones that usually get treated.[26] Hormone treatments, usually in the form of the birth control pill, are frequently prescribed to regulate periods. Birth control pills often alleviate many of the symptoms of PCOS, including acne and mood swings, by reducing or regulating androgen production and restoring normal menstrual bleeding. [27] Other antiandrogens that are sometimes used are medications called spironolactone or cyproterone. [28] For those trying to get pregnant, treatments include medications such as Clomiphene to force ovulation, assisted reproduction techniques, partial ovarian resection, and insulin desensitizing drugs such as Metformin. [29]

Metformin (glucaphage) is also now available and works by suppressing insulin that is produced in the liver. Discuss this option with a knowledgeable endocrinologist familiar with pcos.

Weight loss is also suggested for women with PCOS who are also obese. Obesity, over time, can actually lead to the development of insulin-resistance and diabetes. [30] A diet regimen which restricts calories from fat and carbohydrates, together with a program of physical exercise, can decrease insulin secretion, and help patients lose weight. [31]

Various techniques yield different responses for individuals with PCOS. For example, restrictive diets are difficult to live with so many women, just like typical dieters, give up or go back to regular eating patterns. Some women report great success with drugs such as Metformin while others have reported little or no success.[32] Such reports emphasize that individuals with PCOS need to research their options carefully and may need to try several treatments before reaching success.

Choose rather to punish your appetites than be punished by them.

Tyrius Maximus

Chapter 5
Insulin: The Newest Factor

What is insulin?

Insulin is a hormone that is essential for the metabolism of carbohydrates.

Why should you be concerned with insulin?

- Insulin controls fat build-up and break-down. [33]

- Insulin, the second most powerful salt-retaining hormone next to aldosterone, can produce rapid weight gain from fluid retention rather than excessive intake of calories. [34]

  For those of us with PCOS, this means we suffer from bloating and the accompanying weight gain from water retention. Not only that, but we can put on weight extremely quickly. Of course I probably didn't have to tell you that!

- "High insulin levels may also make the endometrium vulnerable to an enterprising cancer cell." [35]

  Simply put, high levels of insulin increase the risks of developing endometrial cancer. Be sure to see your physician regularly and discuss any concerns you may have at that time.

- PCOS patients with insulin-resistance produce high levels of insulin by the pancreas.[36] This insulin, however, is unable to achieve normal glucose metabolism. The result is that the levels of glucose rise and the body produces yet even more insulin to try to compensate, resulting in hyperinsulinism.[37]

  In everyday terms this means that the insulin in your body is not able to put glucose into the cells the way it is supposed to. The body wrongly thinks that there is a lack of insulin and produces even more, compounding the problem.

What is insulin-resistance?

"In adipose tissue and skeletal muscle, insulin increases glucose uptake. Insulin resistance occurs when, for an average level of insulin in healthy patient, these tissue and muscle do not react normally. It is more difficult for glucose to enter the cells and, to compensate for this defect, more insulin is produced; it forces the glucose into the muscle and adipose tissue." [38]

"As a result, the insulin resistant patient shows both hyperinsulinaemia, due to pancreas overproduction, and hyperglycaemia, caused by the low glucose uptake in tissues."[39] (Hyperinsulinaemia refers to elevated fasting blood insulin levels while hyperglycaemia refers to low blood sugar.) When the pancreas is no longer able to keep up insulin production, glycemia increases and type 2 diabetes can occur.[40]

Make sure that you are tested for diabetes on a regular basis. Most physicians who are familiar with PCOS will suggest these tests to you. If your physician is not familiar with PCOS, you have two options. First, you can educate your physician through materials such as this workbook or printed articles from the Internet. Secondly, you can find a physician who is familiar with the syndrome. In either event, don't hesitate to ask for regular tests.

Causes of insulin-resistance are thought to be:

- "Genetic predisposition;
- Pregnancy;
- Aging;
- Upper abdominal obesity;
- Lifestyle habits such as smoking or lack of exercise; and
- Drugs such as corticosteroids or thiazide diuretics." [41]

How is hyperinsulinemia connected to the other symptoms of PCOS?

Hyperandrogenism is the excessive production of androgens (male hormones) which are often associated with hirsutism, or the excessive growth of hair on the face, chest or abdomen.   Hyperinsulinemia is now thought to cause the hyperandrogenism of PCOS by increasing ovarian androgen production; these high levels of androgenic hormones interfere with the pituitary ovarian axis, leading to increased LH levels, anovulation, amenorrhea, and infertility. [42]

How does this happen?

One theory is that a genetically determined ovarian defect could make the ovary more sensitive to insulin's stimulation of androgen production. [43]   However, researchers are still investigating other possible causes.

What do I do with this new information?

First of all, keep a watchful eye on the research that is now taking place. You can find a lot of information on the Internet and I've included several sources to peruse at the end of this book. When you come upon articles that you think are pertinent to your treatment, print them out and take them to your physician. Do not assume that your physician knows everything about PCOS. Theories and treatments of the condition vary wildly. Ask questions and consider all of your options. The Polycystic Ovary Syndrome Support Group, found at the web address www.pcosupport.org, has a message board where you can communicate with others with PCOS. Find out what works for others and the experiences they have had with different treatments.

Since the first edition of this book in 2001, it has now become more standard practice to prescribe metformin (glucaphage) to control insulin.   Some doctors will prescribe it even if you do not show elevated levels of insulin. Many doctors have reported to me that they have seen significant results with the drug. One endocrinologist said that she was a skeptic until nearly all of her patients taking the drug started having regular periods again and several were able to get pregnant without further fertility treatments. That isn't to say that it is a cure, for it isn't. However, many women find at least some of their symptoms improve. At the very least this should be a conversation piece for you and your doctor. Again, discuss the pros and cons of any risks with your physician - preferably an endocrinologist.

No matter which treatment you choose with your physician, adhering to the sensible diet and exercise techniques in this book will help you to lose weight and lower your insulin levels without medication. Read on to discover how you can begin making lifestyle changes that will begin to improve your health.

One should eat to live, not live to eat.

Benjamin Franklin
1706-1790, American Scientist, Publisher, Diplomat

Chapter 6
Eating to Live

Researchers believe that there is a link to women with PCOS and insulin resistance (your body's ability to use insulin properly). [44] What does this ultimately mean for you? If you have PCOS you likely find yourself craving carbohydrates and sweets. You may feel sluggish when you first wake up in the morning. You may eat a large meal and feel as though you are famished only a few hours later. In fact, it is not unusual for you to feel hungry all the time. You fall into a vicious circle where you crave sweets, eat them, feel sluggish, crave sweets, etc. The more you consume, the less your body can handle. In fact, many women with PCOS will eventually develop Adult Onset Diabetes.

How can you fight this? This chapter addresses two areas: carbohydrate consumption and the basics of eating healthy. Some people, as you are very much aware, can eat anything and not gain a pound. Chances are that you are *not* one of these people. Reconcile yourself that you need to be aware of every morsel of food that goes into your mouth. Read labels. Ingredients are listed in the order of quantity. Therefore, if the second ingredient is sugar or fructose, corn syrup or some other form of sugar, try to avoid it. Look for sugar-free products. A new product on the market is Splenda® which is made from sugar but has no calories. I like to use it to make a low-calorie hot chocolate that tastes great. Splenda® can also be used for baking.

However, be aware of low or non-fat items, which often compensate the decrease in fat by adding sugar. For example, I looked at a Jenny Craig® nutritional bar the other day and noticed that the second ingredient was high fructose corn syrup. Again, read labels. If you must splurge, plan it out. For example, if you know your best friend is having cake at her birthday party, abstain during the week before and allow yourself a few forkfuls. Or you can offer to make a cake yourself with Splenda® and then eat it without worrying about all the processed sugar. Always keep in mind that too much sugar will ultimately result in feeling sluggish, guilty or gaining weight.

Fruits are good sources of sweets, also, but I would moderate those as well. You may have noticed that too much fruit (which contains natural sugars) will make you feel ill. Stock up on vegetables, whole grains and complex carbohydrates. Later in this book I will discuss keeping a journal and noting how foods affect how you feel. Beyond that, make it a habit to plan your meals so that you are in control when you get hungry. Make sure that you have nutritional alternatives when you come home hungry and don't have time to cook a meal. For example, have on hand low-fat and low-sugar cereals and nuts to munch on.

As a regular subscriber to a magazine called *Natural Health*, I recently read that changing eating habits can help those who have type 2 diabetes. The recommendation is to "get 60 percent of calories from fruits, vegetables, and proteins; 20 to 30 percent from complex carbohydrates like grains; and about 15 percent from fat in order to help your insulin work more efficiently."[45] Use the foods you eat to help control your insulin, which in turn controls your metabolism.

A look at carbohydrates:

The subject of carbohydrates has stirred up a national debate. On one side are those who criticize low-carbohydrate diets because of the theory that losing weight is strictly a matter of reducing calories and exercising more. For the population that has no insulin problems, the first theory appears to work. However, as those of us with PCOS know, insulin and blood sugar levels affect how we gain and maintain excess weight. As an answer to this problem, plenty of low-carbohydrate diets have materialized in the last couple of years. Unfortunately, adhering to low-carbohydrate diets can be a gargantuan feat.

Some books recommend eliminating practically all carbohydrates (maintaining only 10 to 30 grams per day) from the diet with no differentiation between "good" and "bad" carbohydrates. What do I mean by good? Although all carbohydrates are actually forms of sugar, complex carbohydrates are released slowly into the bloodstream and provide greater amounts of energy. As you will seen in later examples, a candy bar may have the same amount of carbohydrates as a bowl of cereal but it is ridiculous to think that these foods are acted upon the same way in the body.

For someone with insulin resistance, the shock of the candy bar occurs when the surge of sugar, or glucose, is unable to be processed into the cells by insulin. Afterwards the body produces even more insulin, compounding the problem. The "rejected" sugar then turns into fat, while the blood sugar levels remain elevated. To make matters worse, on the cellular level the cell is crying out that it is hungry because it has been unable to absorb any nutrients. The result? You feel full after eating an enormous amount of candy and junk food but you still feel hungry in spite of the fact that your stomach may actually be hurting because of the amount of food that you have consumed. Sound familiar? Fight back!

Take a focused look at your food labels. Carbohydrates are usually broken down into dietary fiber (which may further be broken down into soluble fiber and insoluble fiber) and sugars. Thus, if I look at a store brand of wheat and barley cereal for a ½ cup serving I may see the following:

Total Carbohydrate	38g
Dietary Fiber	5g
Soluble Fiber	less than 1g
Insoluble Fiber	5g
Sugars	3g
Other Carbohydrates	30g

What does this tell me?

Most labels will list the major breakdowns listed above:

1) Dietary Fiber
2) Sugars
3) Other Carbohydrates

Sugar is what we don't want a lot of, so let's take a look at the total number of carbohydrates as opposed to the amount labeled "sugars."

3 grams per serving seems innocent enough but let's take a further step and figure out what percentage of this product is sugar. The following formula can be used:

(amount of sugar ÷ total carbohydrates) x 100 = percentage of sugar

In this example we can calculate the percentage of the amount of sugars in the serving by dividing 3g (amount listed as sugars) by 38g (total carbohydrates) and multiplying the result to get a rounded total of 8%. I've filled the values in the following formula:

$$(3g \div 38g) \times 100 = .0789 \times 100 = 7.89 = 8\% \text{ when rounded}$$

Therefore, per serving, the cereal consists of only 8% sugar. The remaining 92% consists of dietary fiber and complex carbohydrates. In this case, the cereal is a good choice. As discussed before, complex carbohydrates are broken down more slowly and provide long-range fuel for our bodies. Other sugars tend to be used up quickly and are not usually healthy, especially for those of us with PCOS.

I also like to take a look at the ingredients at the bottom of the nutrition label and verify my findings there. The ingredients for this product are listed as wheat, barley, salt and yeast. That's it. No added sugar. Of course this finding comes as no surprise because it would have yielded a higher number in the breakdown from above.

Let's look at another example. This time we will inspect fruit cocktail. While you certainly want to continue eating fruit as part of a healthy diet, you should also be aware of the high percentage of natural sugars that are found in fruits, especially in concentrates or juices. I selected a fruit cocktail in real fruit juices (no sugar added).

The serving size is listed as ½ cup. To be honest, I could eat at least twice that amount. Keep your own individual serving size in mind when you do your calculations. Be honest. If you ate the whole thing, you need to calculate the ingredients accordingly.

The ingredients in my fruit cocktail example are listed as peaches, water, pears, grapes, pineapple, pear and peach juice concentrates, and colored cherry halves. On the surface this looks like I could eat as much as I want. However, I now know better. I start by looking at the carbohydrate breakdown.

Total Carbohydrate	15g
Dietary Fiber	1g
Sugars	14g

One thing to note first is that fruit cocktail involves skinned fruit as opposed to a fresh piece of fruit. Also, we are consuming juice as well, which though not necessarily unhealthy, is going to have more natural sugar and calories. Once again we apply the following formula to calculate the percentage of sugar.

(amount of sugar ÷ total carbohydrates) x 100 = percentage of sugar

$$(14g \div 15g) \times 100 = .93 \times 100 = 93\%$$

Based on this information, I now realize that there are better sources of fruit. However, if I really love fruit cocktail, then I should keep it in mind for a dessert substitute for candy, cake or other foods with high contents of processed or refined sugars. In this instance, I would be better off eating the fruit with natural sugars. Just don't fool yourself that you are eating the best food choice.

Now, let's look at a really bad food choice, one of those foods that we really love to consume in large quantities. I'll use a name brand chocolate cookie mix as an example. At first glance, you might say that the carbohydrates are no worse than those for the cereal that we looked at earlier. The cereal, if you recall, had 38g of total carbohydrates. In the cookie example, a serving size of two (2) cookies seems like a better choice because it only has 21g of total carbohydrates. The difference is all in sugar content. Intuitively, you already know the truth of this.

We've all had a couple of cookies to ward off a dinner hunger attack as we rush in late from work. Yes, we do get that delightful high. Does it last, though? Of course not. Had we eaten that ½ cup of cereal (used in the example above) then we would have been satisfied a lot longer. Plus, we would have avoided a possible "crash" when the first rush of sugar was placed by a low blood sugar attack (hypoglycemia). Let's continue our investigation.

(amount of sugar ÷ total carbohydrates) x 100 = percentage of sugar

$$(14g \div 21g) \times 100 = .67 \times 100 = 67\%$$

Compared to the cereal example, we can immediately see the benefit of eating the cereal rather than the cookies (in spite of what our taste buds have been trained to want.) The cereal, although higher in total carbohydrates, provides us with a significant lower amount of sugar.

However, based on the previous example, some of you may argue that this cookie example is better than the fruit cocktail example because there is less sugar per serving. While that may be true, you must also consider the inherent nutritional value of the food that you are consuming. Even with a higher percentage of sugar per serving, we know that fruit gives us vitamins and nutrients that the cookies do not. Leave the sweet tooth more healthy alternatives. Examples of these are included in a future chapter.

Other diet considerations:

Avoid fad diets. Weight loss is extremely difficult if you suffer from PCOS. Our metabolism is usually low and we put on weight eating the same amounts or even lesser amounts of food than others. Those of us who have managed to maintain or even lose weight know that it is a *constant* effort. There is no such thing as losing the weight and then continuing back with our normal routine. You must understand that (barring a miracle pill) you will always have to watch everything that you eat and you will always have to exercise in order to keep your weight at an acceptable level. Even though I take glucaphage I still struggle with my weight - although it is much easier since I don't crave food as much and get full more quickly.

There is some research that suggests that patients with PCOS can decrease their insulin by decreasing carbohydrates and fats in our diets.[45] For this book, I have concentrated on slowly changing our eating habits. Feeling deprived doesn't help you to change your eating habits. I suggest starting to slowly eat more complex carbohydrates like whole wheat products and reducing the other carbohydrates. Use the knowledge in this book to research the foods that you consume. In time, when your body has adjusted, you can start eating fewer carbohydrates altogether. My own experience and those of others has shown that extremely limiting carbohydrates can initially make you fatigued and unwilling to exercise.

As daunting as all of this may sound, you can overcome any unhealthy eating habits. Remember, eating healthier and exercising continually will make you look and feel better. You will have greater amounts of energy and will start to feel more in *control*. You *can* make yourself feel better. You can always control how you react to your situation. And control gives you power!

Studies have shown that changing eating lifestyles and weight reduction can lower insulin levels, reduce hyperlipidaemia, lower androgen and luteinizing hormone levels, and improve fertility by restoring regular menstruation and ovulation. [47]

This chapter is designed to help you develop lifelong strategies for healthy eating habits. I've tried to avoid the term "diet" because of the negative connotation many of us have with the word. We've all heard the joke about how the first three letters spell "die." Yet, properly used, diet is simply about the "intake" of food. The concentration should be on putting wholesome foods into the body to provide energy and sustenance.

Have you ever noticed that when you go on a traditional "diet" that food suddenly takes on new meaning? In fact, it is easy to suddenly become obsessed with food when so much of it is forbidden. The impulse is natural and that is why this chapter focuses on the positive aspects of eating. What you want to strive for is a concentration on lifelong health habits. I like to put the emphasis on all the great foods that I can have that will make my body healthier as well. Let me say that I do not endorse a particular "diet" although I do try to limit carbohydrates, especially refined sugars as well as unnecessary fats.

I use the phrase for my new eating habits "eating for life". The idea is to simply eat healthier and think about the good stuff that you can put into your body. For years, even as a child, I would often wake up tired, weak and nauseated for no apparent reason. If I did not eat something within a short period of time, the symptoms would progress to shaking, sweating and occasionally fainting. The symptoms often disappeared after I ate. I should clarify that I am not a diabetic and was confused when my doctors insisted that I was not even a borderline diabetic at the time. I was told to carry around hard candy or crackers in case these episodes continued.

Even before I began taking the glucaphage I found that a healthier diet and the elimination of as much sugar as possible from my diet decreased the attacks. My portions are measured by my hunger level. When I am full, I use the "push-away" method. Simply push your plate away, wrap up any leftovers before you are tempted to eat them, and leave the kitchen.

Most diets do not work because it is against human nature to deprive ourselves of things that we like and/or need. Therefore, our focus must be to train our bodies to crave and like healthier foods. The idea is to train our minds and taste buds to accept healthy food sources rather than the wrong substances we've grown accustomed to packing into our bodies. Remember to start realistically to increase your chances of success. Do not restrict calories too quickly. Do not try to cut out everything cold turkey. This method rarely works.

Two things happen when you cut calories too quickly or severely, depriving yourself of certain foods all at once. First, when calories are cut too quickly, the body reacts as though it is starving. To save itself, your body slows down metabolism. This means your body decreases the number of calories it burns in order to conserve energy, making it even more difficult to lose weight. The second problem is that once we start feel deprived, we start obsessing about food, leading to possible binges. A common effect of people on diets is to lose weight and then gain back all their weight plus a few more pounds once they fall off the diet. There will be times when, in spite of ourselves, we discover that we are gorging on something bad, unable to stop. Afterwards, it is normal to feel guilty and ashamed that we lost control. Learn to take that act as a one-time "slip" and try again the next day. If you give up and let yourself think that it is hopeless then you have let yourself be controlled by your own negativity. Accept the loss of a healthy eating opportunity and then **let it go**.

The next chapter focuses on eating strategies to fight against the ill-effects of PCOS. The purpose of these new strategies is to change your way of thinking about what you put into your body and how you can make simple changes over time to become healthier without going hungry.

Changing our diet is something we choose to do,
not something we are forced to do.
Instead of dreading it, try saying,
"Here's another thing I get to do
to help myself. Great!"

Greg Anderson
Author of "The 22 Non-Negotiable Laws of Wellness"

Chapter 7
Strategies for Healthier Eating

How can you get out of an unhealthy eating cycle? Slowly change eating habits until your body becomes used to less fat and regular processed sugar. Try the suggestions below to convert bad habits into healthy eating:

1. Drink lots of water.

Water makes you feel fuller and keeps you from becoming dehydrated, tired and sluggish.

2. Substitute whole milk with skim milk.

Hate skim milk? You can acquire the new taste. Save a milk carton of the size you ordinarily drink and fill with three quarters whole milk. Add one quarter of skim (non-fat) milk. When you have gotten used to this mixture, add a little more skim milk the next time. Eventually, you will build up to drinking all skim milk without shocking your taste buds. After you have been drinking skim milk for some time, you will find that whole milk tastes unpleasantly thick.

3. Substitute water or juice instead of soft drinks.

Soft drinks contain approximately 8 teaspoons of sugar and contains sodium which causes water retention and bloating.

4.   Avoid high fructose corn syrup.

This thick concentrated sugar is found in a variety of foods. Check labels carefully.

5.   Choose whole fruit over fruit juices.

Fruit juices contain high concentrations of natural sugars and are higher in calories than whole fruit itself.

6.   Substitute vegetable juices for fruit juices.

Tomato juice is a refreshing, tasty alternative to sugary fruit juices. Tomato juice is also filling with fewer calories.

7.   Be aware of fruit "cocktails".

Choose the apple, orange or grapefruit juices over any flavor of "cocktails" and read the label to make sure that it says "no sugar added." The "cocktail" may list sugar as the second ingredient.

8.   Cut and store fresh vegetables in clear plastic bags.

When you want a quick snack you can pull them out in a hurry and nibble on them while you prepare your meals.

9.   Eat five smaller meals per day.

If you can, eat five small meals a day instead of three large meals per day. Going hungry does not make you skinny. In fact, if you skip meals you are more likely to binge eat and consume more calories. Skipping meals can also lead to low blood sugar levels, fatigue and sluggishness.

10. Drink lots of water when you feel bloated.

Bloating and water retention often occurs when there is too much sodium (salt) in the diet. It can also occur with elevated insulin levels. The body retains fluids until it can has enough to flush out excess salts and other impurities. So in spite of the contradiction, increase water consumption when you feel bloated.

11. Use no-sugar added or "low-sugar" spreads.

No sugar added spreads are often artificially sweetened. Low sugar spreads have less sugar than regular spreads.

12. Look for cereals with little or no added sugars.

Not all cereals are alike in terms of healthiness. Check labels for sugar and sodium and compare the carbohydrate breakdowns. If sugar is the second ingredient, don't eat that cereal! Whole wheat brands can be sweetened with   fresh fruit or Splenda®.

13. Check the labels for canned soups.

Try cooking homemade soups. Many canned soups are high in sodium and fat. Soups are simple and inexpensive to make yourself. Just choose fresh vegetables such as celery, cabbage, carrots, and potatoes and add beans or chick peas for a more hearty soup. A can of peeled tomatoes adds nice flavor. Add your favorite spices and allow to simmer for at least an hour.

14. Try cooking sprays when frying.

An innocent looking stir-fry of fresh vegetables can triple in calories if cooking oil is used. Try a cooking spray which has trace amounts of fat in comparison.

15. Substitute the call for vegetable oil with an equal amount of applesauce when baking.

The function of vegetable oil in baking is to add moistness to the recipe. Applesauce is much healthier, has far fewer calories and does the same exact function. This is an excellent way to reduce fat in your favorite dessert.

16. Check your peanut butter label.

Processed peanut butter has lots of sugar. Opt for "natural" peanut butter instead. When you first open a jar of natural peanut butter, you will often find a layer of oil on the top. To reduce the fat, simply pour off the oil and stir the rest up. Natural peanut butter is thicker this way and you may have to adjust to the taste.

17. Read labels on items in the health food stores.

Not all items in health food stores or the health food section of your supermarket are "healthy." Check labels for fat, sugar and sodium content.

18. Buy fat-free or reduced fat cheeses and milk products.

Food manufacturers have improved the taste of their fat-free or reduced fat products. Experiment with brands. Some are better than others. Just check the labels. Some manufacturers add sugar to compensate for less fat.

19. Experiment with spices.

Spices add distinctive flavors without fat or calories. In addition, many of them, including garlic and pepper have been investigated for their health benefits. Cinnamon is said to lower insulin levels. Try them in soups, sprinkle over casseroles or add to vegetables for new flavors.

20. Make your own heathy meals.

Have you ever noticed how paltry some "diet" pre-packaged foods are? I suspect that many have less fat and calories because there is less food.

21. Be creative and serve less high calorie portions.

For example, if you love macaroni and cheese, and are unwilling to give up whole milk or cut down on the butter, add lots of vegetables, such as broccoli, to the final dish or serve small portions of it with other low-calorie items.
You can also serve a rich dessert on a tiny dish so that it looks like it is a large portion but really isn't.

22. Pile your plate first with vegetables.

The "vegetation" part of your dish should take up most of your plate. This will force you to eat smaller portions of starches. If you want seconds, try eating more vegetables instead of breads or starches.

23. Prepare your own lunches.

Even innocent looking take-out platters may have hidden fats and calories. Eating out occasionally is fine, but you will find that preparing your own meals puts *you* in control.

24. Reward yourself for healthy eating habits.

For every candy bar or fattening snack that you avoid, place the appropriate change you would have spent in a jar. When full, treat yourself to something nice, like dance or painting classes or a new pair of sneakers to go walking in!

25. Do not go hungry!

Smaller meals with light snacks will keep your blood sugar level and prevent you from binging while giving you enough energy to exercise as well.

26. Be aware of sugar in your bread.

Many brands of bread have large quantities of processed sugars. I was shocked to discover that sometimes the second ingredient is high fructose corn syrup. Make your own bread or look for nut-flavored breads with less sugar.

27. If you must eat ice cream, choose "no sugar added."

Although eating any ice cream is not the best choice, at least if you are going to splurge make sure that you are consuming as little sugar as possible. These brands typically have at least 1/3 less sugar than their counterparts.

28. If you must eat sweets, eat them in moderation.

Instead of having one big bag of cookies or candy at your fingertips, buy small packages or make up your own smaller versions to prevent compulsive eating. We want to reach a level where we can avoid these sugars altogether. However, it is better to moderate our sweets than to "fast" and then "binge" because we feel so deprived.

29. Buy fat-free, turkey versions of hot dogs.

They have minimal fat and are low in calories.

30. Set realistic goals.

Make realistic changes in your daily eating patterns. Tackle one bad food habit at a time to make yourself feel less deprived. Treat yourself occasionally, in moderation, to the foods that you love the most.

31. Make high fat or high sugar snacks hard to reach.

I once had a friend who curbed his credit card usage by locking the cards in a box, wrapping a chain around the box, locking the chain, then putting the whole contraption in a difficult place to reach in the basement. The cards were so difficult to get to that he often decided against using them. Use this rationale to make poor snack choices inaccessible. Find a high cabinet where you must get a chair or ladder to gain access. Put cookies, high fat chips, etc. in sealed containers and push them to the back wall. At the very least you will get a workout trying to get to them!

32. Using a small plate to make portions seem larger.

A large plate with just a little bit of food can appear unsatisfying. However, a well-heaped small plate (with the same amount of food) can seem very satisfying.

33. Take a notepad with you when you go shopping.

As you read labels, write down the brands that are low in sugar and fat. The next time that you go shopping, you can refer to your notes and reduce your browsing time.

34. Chart your progress.

Keep a journal that details the *positive* aspects of your new healthy lifestyles. Find something good every day to write about, even if it is a simple thing such as "I ate one more piece of fruit today than yesterday. Tomorrow I will try to add another vegetable to my diet." Working towards a goal is easier if we can see achievements along the way.

35. Enlist a friend or join a support group.

Changing lifestyle habits are difficult. Having support increases the chance of success in modifying eating habits and activity level. A listing of resources is included at the back of this book.

36. If a support group does not exist in your area, start one yourself.

There is no need to wait for someone to start up a group in your area if one is lacking. Post messages on e-mail bulletin boards on sites such as www.pcosupport.org or put up fliers in community areas such as the library, post office, or supermarket bulletin boards.

37. Decrease sodium in your diet.

Check labels and opt for other spices to flavor foods.

Remember that a little change every day is better than a lot of changes at once that don't last. Take these suggestions and tailor them to meet your own individual needs. You are the most important factor in the equation. Just realize that you can do *anything* that you feel that you *must* do, an idea by Dan Millman, author of *Everyday Enlightenment.* I have certainly found that thought to be true.

Nothing lifts me out of a bad mood better than a hard workout on my treadmill. It never fails. To us, exercise is nothing short of a miracle.

Cher
1946-, American Actress, Director, Singer

Chapter 8
Exercise

You were probably hoping that I wouldn't bring this up. I can already hear the excuses. After all, you have a job and then you get home and have to fix dinner. Before you know it you are too tired to even crawl to bed, let alone do some exercises. Or maybe you just hate exercise? Or you already exercise but don't see any results? Keep trying!

In order to fight against PCOS you will have to make exercise a priority. You will have to make it just as important as bathing, brushing your teeth, or eating. Find something that you love to do, whether it be walking or swimming or playing tennis. Whatever routine you pick, make sure that it involves a physical activity that you can do every day. For those with PCOS, it is important that exercise be a necessary habit.

Why exercise?

First, 20 to 30 minutes of aerobic activity 2 to 3 times a week helps you not only lose weight, but it helps your body use insulin more efficiently.[48] Exercise makes you stronger, increases your energy, increases your metabolism, tones your body, adds years to life expectancy, and motivates you to eat better. After you've walked five miles or pedaled a stationary bike for thirty minutes you will find yourself a lot less willing to "ruin" your workout by eating junk food. And if you are like me, apt to eat the most when you feel the worst about your body, exercise will start to change your image and help you to get out of those bad habits and associations. Exercise is vital for a variety of reasons. In addition to helping you lose weight, exercise can:

- Build endurance and stamina
- Improve self-confidence
- Firm up your body
- Increase metabolism
- Help you sleep more soundly
- Increase your energy levels
- Increase flexibility
- Increase coordination
- Increase life expectancy
- Be fun!

When establishing your exercise regime, be sure to include strength training. Why strength training? The more muscle you have, the higher your metabolism will be. In essence, muscle burns more calories. That means that the more you exercise, the less diminished your meals have to be. In addition, muscle burns calories even while you rest or sleep.

I personally like pushups and situps as part of my strength training. My favorite form of aerobic exercise is swimming because I love the water and can't feel myself sweat. Decide what is best for you. Most importantly, however, pick something that looks and feels *fun!* Find your niche.

There are two important things to remember when starting an exercise program:

1) Check with your physician, especially if you have illnesses or conditions that might be adversely affected by increased activity level.

2) Choose an activity that you sincerely enjoy.

If you start an exercise program for the sole sake of losing weight, chances are you are not going to like it. Running may burn more calories, but if you absolutely hate to get up and run in the morning, how long are you realistically going to stick with it? There are many fun activities that you can choose to have fun and get in shape. However, remember that you need to try to do *some* sort of exercise on a daily basis. Some questions to ask yourself as you choose an activity are:

- Do I like team sports?
- Do I like to work out individually?
- Do I love getting outdoors?
- Do I love activities I can do in my own home?
- Do I like competition?
- Do I like working out at my own pace?
- Can I afford gym fees?
- Do I have an exercise partner?
- Will I have family support?
- Do I need to see a physician before starting?
- Do I have any physical limitations? (Bad knee, etc.)
- What physical activity do I really love doing?
- If I exercised previously, why did I stop?
- Is there an outdoor or indoor track I have access to?
- Would my partner or spouse exercise with me?
- Are there physical activities that I can participate in with my family as a whole?

Consider the answers to the above questions as you contemplate the following exercise options. Remember that you can mix and match activities. For example, go to a gym 3 days a week, take a swimming class 2 days a week and use your treadmill the other 2 days. Keeping active throughout the week will keep you energized.

Just remember that you need to make exercise a *daily* habit.

JOINING A GYM

Positive aspects:

- Meet and work out with new people
- Social atmosphere conducive to setting goals
- Safe environment

Negative aspects:

- Intimidating for some individuals
- Costly with initiation and monthly fees
- Must have discipline to get to the gym

WALKING OR RUNNING

Positive aspects:

- Only the expense of a good pair of shoes
- Can schedule your routine any time you like
- No travel necessary if you have a safe running area in the neighborhood
- If you have a track in the neighborhood you can meet with others

Negative aspects:

- Must always be cautious when walking or running alone

- Never walk or run at night or in unknown neighborhoods
- Harder to stay disciplined if you are not working out with others

VIDEO WORKOUTS

Positive aspects:

- Exercise from comfort of home
- Work at your own pace
- Use the rewind button to master routines
- Inexpensive
- Variety - Stock up on several sessions
- Your partner, friends or children can join you
- Flexible workout times

Negative aspects:

- No instructor oversight
- Requires discipline to work out alone

PURCHASING EXERCISE EQUIPMENT

Positive aspects:

- Control your own schedule
- Avoid commuting to a gym

- In the long-term, investing in equipment is less expensive than enrolling at a gym
- Improved chances of continued workout if you have the equipment in your own home
- Great for those who are too intimidated or embarrassed to work out at the gym
- Others in the home can also participate

- Some exercises, like walking on a treadmill, can be done while you are watching television or listening to music

Negative aspects:

- Depending on the equipment, initial expense can be costly
- No instructor oversight
- Self-discipline to increase repetitions and intensity
- Many people buy equipment and then neglect to use it

JOINING AN ATHLETIC TEAM OR GROUP

Positive aspects:

- Activities and team sports can be fun
- Great way to meet others
- A good team will provide support and encouragement
- Competition provides incentive and excitement

Negative aspects:

- In order to get exercise on a daily basis, you need to make sure that you do some other type of exercise on the days when your are not participating in a sport
- Must make sure that everyone gets to play. If you get "benched" a lot you are obviously not getting a workout
- Intimidating if you have never been particularly good at team sports

TAKING DANCE LESSONS

Positive aspects:

- Dancing is fun and healthy

- Music can sweep you away, making you forget that you are burning calories
- Physical activity in a friendly safe environment
- Socialize with others

Negative aspects:

- Lessons can be expensive
- Must be willing to try new things
- Some people may be intimidated or embarrassed because of weight issues

TAKING MARTIAL ARTS

Positive aspects:

- Martial arts build character and confidence
- Coordination is improved
- Self-discipline is taught
- Fun activity
- Competition at higher levels

Negative aspects:

- Lessons can be expensive
- Must be willing to take risks and try new things
- Some people may be intimidated or embarrassed because of weight issues

Get started!

Now that you have some ideas, why not get started on an exercise program right away.

Pick several activities that you would like to try.

1. _____

2. _____

3. _____

4. _____

Are these activities realistic in terms of how much time you have and what type of activity you feel most comfortable doing? If so, then plan something for today.

Today I will:

1. _____

2. _____

3. _____

4. _____

If you want to join a team or take dance lessons, for example, stop now and find the number in your local phone book for a soccer club, tennis club or dance studio. Find out about any dues or fees and calculate if they fit into your budget. If you want to start walking or running, determine if you have the appropriate shoes.

Things I need:

1. _____

2. _____

3. _____

Once you are prepared, then get started as soon as possible. Do not wait until next week. Some people think that they must start an activity on a Monday, for example. Monday comes and goes and now they must wait for the *next* Monday. Do not delay your exercise program for silly reasons like this. You can start any day of the week. Unless you are enrolling in a structured program, it does not matter when you begin. Begin **today!**

Lots of people limit their possibilities by giving up easily.
Never tell yourself this is too much for me.
It's no use. I can't go on. If you do you're licked,
and by your own thinking too. Keep believing
and keep on keeping on.

Norman Vincent Peale
1898-1993, American Christian Reformed Pastor,
Speaker, Author

Chapter 9
Pregnancy

Infertility is one of the most disconcerting and frustrating aspects of PCOS. If you are trying to get pregnant, you should discuss your options with your physician, preferably a reproductive endocrinologist. If you have already tried to get pregnant, you may find that you have entered a very baffling world where your doctor may be just as perplexed as you are. Find a doctor who is familiar with Polycystic Ovary Syndrome and continue to do your own research.

When I first discovered, at the age of twenty, that I would be facing the problems of infertility, I was stunned. I had always assumed a certain logical order of events in my life. I would finish college, get married and have a family. To not have children had never entered my imagination. Today, as a newlywed ready to begin a family I am finally trying to conceive. However, I accept the fact that one day adoption may be my best alternative. I have met other women who face infertility and their experiences have taught me that trying to conceive can place a devastating emotional burden on a couple.

If you have PCOS, and have not been able to get pregnant, get all the information that you can from your physician about what your alternatives are. Keep in mind that conceiving is not an easy process. Prepare yourself to answer the following challenging questions:

1)   What time frame will I establish for trying to conceive?

2)   Does my partner agree with my time frame for trying to conceive?

3)   Do I have complete emotional and physical support for trying to conceive by assisted reproduction, if such means become necessary?

4)   Am I fully aware of possible side affects caused from taking drugs in order to conceive?

5)   Will my insurance cover all the medical procedures that may become necessary in trying to conceive? Note that states differ in their policies regarding coverage of fertility assistance. Check your individual health insurance policy and check out others as well.

6)   If attempts at conception are unsuccessful, am I comfortable with the thought of adoption?

7)   How does my partner feel about adoption?

8)   Have I educated myself about new treatments for fertility?

9)   Is my physician aware of new treatments for fertility?

10)   Have I fully researched all possibilities and alternatives?

I have known women who have been trying, unsuccessfully, for years to conceive. They have tried almost everything in the book - from daily shots to in vitro fertilization. The toll is great and often creates a strain on a marriage. The more informed both you and your partner are in the beginning of the process, the better your chances are of keeping your sanity and your tempers intact. My husband and I have decided that we will try for about a year to get pregnant. We have been hoping that the glucaphage will help us to conceive naturally. At the end of nine months of trying we will take the next step and our doctor will be prescribing Clomid, a drug that stimulates the ovary to produce eggs. Because Clomid usually works within the first three months or so - if it is going to work at all - we will only take it for that length of time before seeking the advice of a fertility specialist. If we are still not pregnant then we will take about a year and then start the adoption process. We have decided not to do any extensive fertility treatment such as IVF. This is our personal decision and yours may be different.

Do your own research and decide what is best for you and your husband.

When you are trying, you should have candid conversations with your spouse and determine what is best for you. Explore all alternatives but don't feel compelled to *have* to try every single one. Ultimately, only you, your spouse and doctor can determine the best way to go forward. Be prepared, however, to do your research. Make sure that you are familiar and knowledgeable about any associated risks. The Polycystic Ovary Syndrome Support Page (www.pcosupport.org) is a great place to find stories and experiences from others.

If you make the unconditional commitment
to reach your most important goals,
if the strength of your decision is sufficient,
you will find the way and the power to achieve your goals.

Robert Conklin
American Teacher, Author

Chapter 10
New Treatments

What are the new possibilities for treating PCOS?

In the past, women such as myself were told that PCOS was "just an infertility problem." We were put on birth control, perhaps prescribed drugs for the excessive hair and acne and sent on our merry way. Those times are changing, albeit somewhat slowly.

Some promising new treatments are standard medicines used for treating adult-onset diabetes; these drugs lower serum insulin concentrations and are in the form of metformin (Glucophage 500 or 850 mg three times a day with meals) and troglitazone (Rezulin 400 mg once a day). [49]

Additionally, INS-1 is a drug researched in a study conducted by Daniela Jakubowicz, MD, at the Hospital Clinicas de Caracas in Venezuela in collaboration with John Nestler, MD, at the Medical College of Virginia. [50]

Another insulin-sensitizing drug is Rosiglitazone. Rosiglitazone, to be marketed under the brand name Avandia, is in the final stages of pre-approval testing and its function is to make muscle tissue more sensitive to the body's own insulin. [51] Rosiglitazone, a chemical relative of troglitazone (Rezulin) does not appear to cause the rare but serious liver problems of troglitazone and is also more potent than troglitazone, making it effective at a lower dose. [52]

How effective are these treatments?

Both metformin and Rezulin medications have been shown to reverse the endocrine abnormalities associated with PCOS within two or three months and can result in decreased hair loss, diminished facial and body hair growth, normalization of elevated blood pressure, regulation of menses, weight loss and normal fertility. [53] Researchers have even seen pregnancies result in less than two months in women who conceived in the very first ovulatory menstrual cycle.[54]

A study of 16 non-diabetic PCOS patients performed by Charles J. Glueck, MD at the Cholesterol Center, Jewish Hospital, in Cincinnati Ohio, indicated that metformin therapy lowered insulin, reducing the levels of plasminogen activator inhibitor activity (PAI-1). [55] PAI-1 is an independent risk factor for heart attack and stroke because it reduces the ability of the body to dissolve blood clots. [56]

The findings of another clinical study were presented at the 58th scientific sessions of the American Diabetes Association, showing that the drug INS-1 was effective in producing ovulation in women with PCOS.[57] 86% of the women treated with INS-1 ovulated compared to only 27% of women in the placebo group of the randomized, double-blind, placebo-controlled study which involved 44 obese women with PCOS. [58] In addition, there were significant decreases in serum insulin and testosterone levels among women who received INS-1. [59]

In a Rosiglitazone study of 493 type-2's (adult onset-diabetes) participants who received 8mg of the drug showed a 76 mg/dl drop in blood glucose more than those participants receiving a placebo. [60] 40 percent of the participants taking the Rosiglitazone had blood glucose levels of less than 140 mg/dl after the end of the 26-week study.[61] The results of the study were presented at an American Diabetes Association meeting in Chicago. [62] The benefits of insulin reduction for the patient are relief from hunger and carbohydrate cravings, a decrease in elevated triglycerides, hypertension relief, and increased levels of the neurotransmitter serotonin, which has a calming affect and improves sleep patterns. [63]

Are these medications safe?

The safety of Rezulin, known generically as troglitazone, has recently been questioned after being linked to at least 40 cases of acute liver failure, resulting in 28 deaths, prompting a panel of doctors to recommend that while the drug's benefits outweigh any risks, the drug was too risky to be used alone, an important implication for sufferers of PCOS who would generally use the drug alone. [64]

Metformin appears safe when given to non-diabetic patients and does not lower blood sugar.[65] Side effects during the first week of taking the medication include upset stomach or diarrhea.[66] Such side affects can be minimized for those taking metformin if the dosage is begun with one pill daily for the first week, followed by and increase to two pills per day the second week.[67] Patients like myself have found that taking the medication with food or milk greatly decreases the likelihood of upset stomach.

Metformin should be given cautiously, however, to patients with renal function because they are at a higher risk for a rare side effect called lactic acidosis. [68]

Data for the safety of use during pregnancy is not conclusive and the general recommendation is that the medication be avoided during pregnancy until more definitive data on the safety of such usage is determined. [69]

There are also the implications of what happens when PCOS is not treated effectively. Limited success by traditional treatments such as weight loss diets, ovulation medications, and anti-androgen medications (birth control pills, spironolactone, flutamide or finasteride) treat only the symptoms and not the root of the problem. The risks of developing diabetes, increased risk of heart attack and stroke, and endometrial cancer must also be weighed when considering other options. [70]

A growing number of researchers feel that sufficient evidence justifies the clinical use of insulin-sensitizing medications in the treatment of women with PCOS. [71]

Where can I get some of these diabetic treatments?

At the time of this writing, the FDA has not approved the use of diabetic medications for the general use by women with PCOS, although several clinical trials are underway. Both the safety and effectiveness must be determined before the FDA gives its approval.

However, doctors are able to prescribe such drugs as glucaphage as "off-label" use. You may have to search to find such a doctor but the practice is gaining acceptance, particularly among endocrinologists. Many medications are also being tested in clinical trials. To obtain information about clinical trials in your area, visit the Polycystic Ovary Syndrome Support Page. Before beginning any clinical trial or starting any new medication, however, do your research. The Polycystic Ovary Syndrome Support Page links to a discussion board where you can ask others which medications they have tried and what the results have been. Some experienced relief when starting the medications and others seemed to feel that their condition had worsened.

Individual experiences vary greatly and you should consider your options carefully, especially if you are taking experimental medication that has not been approved by the FDA. No one can make the decision for you; however, you should realize that there are risks associated with many of these drugs. I've been very happy thus far with my use of metformin (glucaphage). However, each woman must weigh the alternatives with her physician and decide on her own best course of action.

**Our greatest weakness lies in giving up.
The most certain way to succeed is always
to try just one more time.**

Thomas A. Edison
1847-1931, American Inventor, Entrepreneur, Founder of GE

Chapter 11
Finding Meaning and Inner Strength

Fighting PCOS can be an emotional struggle as well as a physical struggle. Yet, we can find meaning and inner strength to pull us through. We have all heard stories about people on their death beds and how doctors will say that the patient has lost the will to live. I believe that in all illnesses, our "will" helps determine, or at least helps shape, our well-being.

What does this have to do with PCOS?

PCOS is a complex condition that demands much patience, tenacity, fortitude, optimism and self-assurance. Any medical problem can prove difficult. The patient with PCOS struggles with weight issues, self-esteem, mood swings from hormonal imbalances, the frustrations of infertility, the fears of developing endometrial cancer, the apprehension of developing heart disease or diabetes, the anger at having all of these various symptoms and not always being able to fight back effectively.

Often there are feelings of being all alone in fighting this condition. Though we may meet others struggling with the same physical symptoms, it becomes easy to feel down about what is happening to our bodies. Writing this book has been one way in which I can find meaning to having PCOS. Sharing my story may help someone else.

If you could find a way to make something positive happen because of your condition, think of how that would help you. Rape victims, for example, often talk about how talking to teenagers often helps them find meaning and understanding in their own lives. They take a tragic experience and use that experience to gain new insights and to educate others.

Having a serious medical condition also forces us to approach life in a very different manner than we may have approached it before. For example, having children does not seem like such a miracle until you have been told that you are medically infertile and will probably experience many difficulties in trying to conceive. How different children seem then! They become rare gifts and we may feel punished not to deserve the same gifts as others.

To become bitter about such prospects is not uncommon; how easy it would be to feel sorry for ourselves. We think about all the teenagers who seem to get pregnant so easily; we consider the large numbers of abortions performed each year; we agonize facing the possibility that children may not be meant for us.

Yet, to give in to those feelings of helplessness, disparity and even anger, would be to yield yet another part of our life to PCOS.

What can we do? I believe that we need to:

1)   Experience all the negative feelings that occur without trying to suppress them and

2)   Let them go.

Let them go?

I know. I know. Easier said than done. However, holding grudges, even grudges against an illness, can be further debilitating to your body. The power of positive thinking and feeling can do wonders.

I once read an article in a magazine that talked about how important it was when you were at home with a bad cold or the flu to get dressed and put on your makeup. At the time, I thought that the article was ridiculous. Since then, however, I've tried out the technique. My experience is that the magazine article was right. On days when I stayed at home, not showering, wearing no makeup, not bothering to wash my hair, I felt sick *and* depressed.

In addition, to my sore throat and other bodily aches and pains, I found that I sat around feeling sorry for myself. On the other hand, on the days when I forced myself into the shower, put on my makeup, found myself a funny movie on television or video, my symptoms did not seem as bad. I'm sure you've had similar experiences.

What I'm getting at is that even though you may suffer from PCOS, you do not have to give in to all the negative emotions that come with it. Use whatever means you have to make sure that your mental health and well-being are not sabotaged by your condition.

How can I stay positive?

You are the best person to determine what "tricks" work for you staying in a positive frame of mind. I've listed some of my own favorites next.

- Listening to upbeat music

- Calling a good friend who makes you laugh

- Watching a funny movie

- Taking a hot bubble bath in candlelight

- Reading one of my favorite books

- Taking a long walk with my walkman keeping me company

- Making a gift package for someone else

- Sorting through cute baby pictures of myself and my siblings - always good for a few laughs!

- Cooking a new recipe and sharing it with friends

- Turning out all the lights in my room and dancing (I wouldn't want anyone to see me!)

- Going shopping for new clothes

- Surfing the Internet just for fun

- E-mailing friends

- Writing a real handwritten letter as a special treat for a friend

- Sending e-mail cards to friends - "just because"

- Arrange to meet an old friend for lunch and a movie

- Go to an art gallery or museum (with a friend or even by yourself)

- Visit your local park

- Take a day trip and go somewhere you don't usually visit

- Go for a swim or get some other type of exercise

What you decide to do makes no difference really. The idea is that you take the emphasis off yourself and concentrate on the world around you. It is simplistic but it works.

Always remember that there are support groups and others who understand you as well. Visit the Polycystic Ovary Syndrome Support page when you need solace.

In essence, if we want to direct our lives,
we must take control of our consistent actions.
It's not what we do once in a while that shapes
our lives, but what we do consistently.

Anthony Robbins
1960-, American Author, Speaker,
Peak Performance Expert / Consultant

Chapter 12
A Lifestyle Journal

Why a lifestyle journal?

You may be wondering why I entitled this chapter a lifestyle journal or why I'm insinuating that you need any sort of journal at all. Women with PCOS have such complex issues surrounding their health, making it difficult to keep track of what we are doing with our bodies, what works well and what makes us feel ill. We must keep track of our hormonal medications, if we are taking them, as well as monitoring how our diet and exercise affects our weight, energy levels, and moods. When my blood sugar level dropped in the past, I often became lightheaded, disoriented and cranky. I noticed that when I stopped eating sugary snacks during the day, I suddenly stopped having afternoon cravings. In addition, my energy levels surged. What was going on here? Depending on how I treated my body, my mood and energy levels experienced differing effects.

Will everyone experience the same effects as I did? Of course not. We all have different bodies, different chemistries and different levels of hormones and insulin. There is not a single "one size fits all" approach to feeling your best. That is where a lifestyle journal comes in. A lifestyle journal can be a notebook or diary or even a large bulletin board where each day lists the foods you have eaten, the times you have eaten, whether you took the appropriate medication, if any, the exercise you performed and, most importantly, what effect each had on your energy level and general feeling of overall health.

Whether your lifestyle journal is simple or complex makes no difference. The important thing is to discover what works for your body and what works against your body. YOU are the best person for this job! Write in your journal **every** day, not just on the days when you feel like you did well. Those bad days will show you how your unhealthy eating habits can control you, if you let them.

Why not just start immediately on a diet?

Diets are not normally tailored to special needs of individuals. Depending on the diet, you are asked to reduce calories and eat specific foods. For many healthy individuals this *sometimes* works. Often it does not.

What's the problem?

The problem is that we all have very different eating patterns, daily food and calorie intakes, different metabolisms and different exercise levels. In essence, we all have differing needs and concerns. To complicate matters, the PCOS patient may not be eating a lot of calories in the first place. It is highly likely that she may be eating the same amounts or even fewer calories than her healthy and slim counterparts. If she is insulin-resistant then her body can not metabolize properly and use up the glucose that she intakes. PCOS is associated with obesity. It is important to realize that if you are obese, it is a physical problem. You are not lazy or a glutton. You must learn, however, how to eat the foods that allow your body to function the best that it can.

What can I do?

You should realize that you must work harder at losing weight or maintaining your weight. Given that, accept the challenge and *move on.* First, establish exactly what your eating habits are. I suggest beginning with what I call an **Existing Intake Journal**. This journal documents your eating habits: what time you eat, what you typically eat, and how these foods make you feel. Be honest. If you eat donuts every morning, be honest about it. Also include "just a taste" items. How many of us have simply "tasted" the cookie dough as we were making cookies for the office? Write it down!

This manual is not about temporary diets. We want to strive towards making lifelong eating habits that will make us look and feel our best.

The **Existing Intake Journal** is a beginning. It shows you where you are on the map to well-being. After you get your bearings, you will begin to chart your progress as you work towards your goals. Once you have established any bad eating habits, you can then work on *gradually* changing those habits to more healthy ones. Following is a sample of an approach that you can use to construct your journal.

Sample Journal Entry

Friday, March 19, 1999

Lost control and ate one quarter of a bag of candy that I purchased to make Easter baskets for my nephews. Result: Could not stop myself. Felt out of control. Intense cravings for sweets that was not satisfied even after I finished off the bag. Later I felt tired and sluggish. Did not feel like exercising. Felt like: "What's the point after sabotaging my good eating habits?" Later in the evening after eating regular dinner, I had surge of energy. Stayed up late but snacked during the night on starchy foods like sweet potatoes.

Saturday, March 20, 1999

Had difficulty waking up this morning. Felt tired and weak. Took several glucose tablets in attempt to raise my blood sugar level but could not get rid of sluggishness. Took a long nap for several hours during the day. Had difficulty waking up. Felt better after eating a normal meal and avoiding excess sugar for the remainder of the day and evening. Had burst of energy late in the evening. Stayed up late again but this time did not eat anything before I slept. Woke up tired but not sick. Was very hungry but did not have associated nausea.

Analyzing the journal.

The next step is to analyze the weekly journal. I can not overemphasize the need to spend a lot of time and effort at this step. The keys to changing your lifestyle eating habits are:

1)   Recognizing current healthy habits;
2)   Identifying habits that need improvement; and
3)   Substituting new healthier habits

This approach seems incredibly easy; yet, most people do not stop to consider what they are placing into their bodies on a day to day basis. I was shocked to discover that I rarely ate fruits and vegetables. I make a point of including these items on a grocery list before I go shopping. The above samples are typical of some of my own pitfalls. I have included them, as well as an analysis, to demonstrate how I tackled my own faulty eating habits.

Analysis #1: (journal entry dated Friday, March 19)

I should know better. Next time package up any "gifts" before I'm tempted to eat them. Or make myself a "gift" bag containing only one or two pieces of the candy. For me, though, it is easier not to eat any at all than to control how much I eat. Also, this was a result of poor organization and preparation. I did not have adequate other foods to snack on such as cut-up vegetables.

Analysis #2: (journal entry dated Saturday, March 20)

Eating sweets late at night always makes me feel tired and sluggish the next morning. Again, this was a problem caused by poor planning. Faced with chocolates and nothing else to snack on, the most strong-willed of us will weaken and eat the chocolate. The fact that I felt better after eating a normal meal shows me how sensitive my body is to having complex carbohydrates. Not eating during the night seemed to positively affect how I felt the next day.

What next?

Now take the information you have gathered and use it to begin a healthier lifestyle. Your journal entries should have indicated the problem areas that you need to work on. Now you need to establish goals and maintain a diet journal.

Establishing Goals

What goals have you determined that you need to take? Do you need to include more fruits and vegetables in your diet? Do you need to make low-fat substitutions? Do you need to substitute an artificial sweetener in your coffee in the morning rather than sugar? Take a moment to fill in a list of goals in the section provided below.

Goals to a healthier diet and lifestyle:

1. _____

2. _____

3. _____

4. _____

5. _____

Maintaining a Diet Journal

After you have determined your goals, you can begin your new diet journal. You will write down your goals for the day either the night before or early in the morning. Establishing goals is an important step to achieving success.

I would suggest taking the goals on a **day by day** basis. Do not make this process too complex. Also, do not try to achieve more goals per day than is realistic. If you have been eating steak and eggs for breakfast every day, eat out in fast food restaurants on a daily basis and have midnight snacks of cookies with milk every night, do not go cold turkey all at once or you will drive yourself crazy and your body will feel as though it is going in shock. Remember that these are lifetime, lifestyle changes. The more realistic the goals you set, the better the chance you have of making long-term changes.

Also take the time to indicate the exact times of your meals. Timing between meals can be crucial in gaining control of binge eating as well as general well-being and energy levels. I noticed that eating late at night made me feel ill and sluggish in the morning. Skipping meals makes me tired, cranky and nauseated. Eating more frequently (i.e.

several smaller "meals" during the day) optimizes my energy level and seems to control my blood sugar levels.

Be sure to include a section on "how I felt?" It is important to connect the types of foods you are eating and when you are eating them to how they make you feel.

Strength does not come from physical capacity. It comes from an indomitable will.

Mahatma Gandhi
1869-1948, Indian Political, Spiritual Leader

Chapter 13
Self Empowerment

The purpose of this book has been to enhance self-awareness of factors that can alleviate or aggravate many of the symptoms and conditions associated with PCOS. Knowledge can help change your lifestyle and fosters a sense of control and self-empowerment. When I first learned of the many negative associations of PCOS, I felt out of control and helpless. How could I lose weight or maintain a strong healthy body when I was faced with the possibility of developing diabetes, endometrial cancer or heart disease? What chance did I have when faced with these obstacles? What could I do if my body produced too much insulin, slowing down my metabolism and making it extremely difficult to lose weight? Why not just accept the facts and let what might happen, happen?

What I eventually realized was that I do have control. Maybe I can not change the fact that I have PCOS. Maybe I can not wave a magic wand and make my body thin like the models I see in magazines. What I can do, however, is to take control of those aspects of my lifestyle that can and do make a difference. How I feel about myself, how strong I am, and how I fight the odds of developing diabetes and heart disease can be controlled by changing lifelong eating and exercise habits.

This process is not an easy one. Habits are not changed overnight. I will always struggle with certain foods that I want to eat more of than I should. I will always have to exercise to maintain an ideal body weight.

Commitment

To help me stay on track and to stay focused on my goals I have developed the following vows to stay committed without being too hard on myself. I hope that they help you, also, as you struggle with this condition.

I Vow to:

- Exercise because it makes me feel good.

- Eat healthy foods for energy and to fight PCOS.

- Start each day as a new beginning.

- Never "beat up" myself when I gain a pound or eat the wrong foods. I will try harder the next day.

- Continue to educate myself about PCOS.

- Spreak frankly with my doctor about issues of PCOS.

- Eat more fresh vegetables.

- Seek out nutritious meals and recipes.

- Control my diet instead of letting my diet control me.

- Stay positive. I will not let PCOS define my life's happiness.

- Use my experience to help others.

Self-Empowerment

Who better to create a sense of power than YOU? You alone hold the knowledge of your desires, fears, wants and needs. The first step to becoming self-empowered is to decide what your goals are. What will it take for you to feel a sense of power and control in your life? Some of you reading this may be severely overweight. Maybe you feel, as I did, that food dictates your behaviors. Perhaps you want to have more energy and participate in more activities. Or maybe you are not happy with the size or condition of your body. Only you can decide what your goals are.

Take a moment now and write these goals down in the spaces provided below. This step is extremely important. How can you work towards achieving better health if you haven't made a commitment to even yourself? Be as specific as possible. Don't just say "eat better" or "eat more healthy." Instead, write down exactly what aspect you are trying to improve. For example, one of your goals may be to reduce the sugar in your daily diet. Another goal may focus on exercise. Again, be specific. Instead of saying "exercise more" you might write that your goal is to be able to run three miles within the next six months.

1. _____

2. _____

3. _____

4. _____

5. _____

Now take a moment and think about why you feel so strongly about these goals. In order to stick to a regime that will bring you closer to achieving a goal, you *must* feel strongly about that goal. For me, I decided that my overall health was extremely important to me. I feel very strongly about reducing my chances of developing diabetes and heart disease. The grim reality of a 40% chance of developing diabetes frightened me. My reason for wanting to increase my overall health gave me motivation to set and achieve several goals.

Take a moment and write down a reason for achieving each of your goals. Remember, the stronger the reason, the greater the motivation for achieving your goals.

1. _____

2. _____

3. _____

4. _____

5. _____

Now that you are motivated to accomplish the goals that you have set for yourself, you need to establish workable steps for achieving those goals. Keep in mind that the best way to achieve a goal is to break it down into manageable steps. Let's say that one of your goals is to limit sugar in your daily diet. The following steps could help you making this goal achievable. In this example I found that each step could also be broken down into further steps, so I have used indents to show subsections.

1. Identify sugary foods in my daily diet.

    Keep a daily food journal
    Read food labels

2. Find appropriate substitutes

    Find new recipes
    Revamp current recipes

3. Enlist the help of friends and family

    Make decision and goals known
    Ask for help in finding new recipes
    Request alternatives at family events
    Ask for moral support
    Share great recipes!

4. Chart your progress

5. Celebrate successes (not with food!)

With these new tools, you will be able to take control of your health and well-being. Remember you can do anything you decide to do. If you walk away from reading this book with nothing else, just remember that you have two choices. You can either let PCOS control your life or you can learn to control your health and well-being through lifestyle changes.

Take ACTION! Don't let PCOS control you.

Start NOW! Set goals and change those habits. The only person you are doing this for is yourself.

Although there is a great deal of controversy
among scientists about the effects of ingested food
on the brain, no one denies that you can change your
cognition and mood by what you eat.

Arthur Winter

Chapter 14
Sample Dishes

The following meal samples below are simply nutritious meals that will help guide you to eating better without going hungry. Many of the items include recipes.

Breakfast Items:

I find that eating sugary foods, including many fruits, in the morning, has a tendency to make me feel fatigued and nauseated. In fact, depending on what and when I ate my last meal I may wake up literally starving. Below are some of my favorite breakfast items.

- Fat-Free Turkey bacon

    (Use cooking spray to make it crisp in the frying pan.)

- Vegetable Omelets

    (tomatoes, onions, and bell peppers are all good choices)

- Fruit Filled Pancakes

    I love to use bananas or blueberries to make extra special pancakes. Use a reduced fat or fat-free pancake mix and prepare as directed. When the mix is ready, add mashed ripe bananas or fresh blueberries. Both work fine.

Be aware of some fruits with a high water content. If experimenting with peaches, for example, use less water in the batter mixture. Blueberry pancakes are my favorites. The blueberries will "explode" as the pancake cooks, making them warm and delicious. Try using a reduced sugar syrup or, even better, try them with a non-fat, sugar-free whipped topping for a special treat. Fat-free turkey bacon goes well with these. Because you are getting sugars from the fruit in the pancakes, I would suggest drinking skim milk or a non-juice beverage such as water, tea or coffee, with this meal.

Other items I like for breakfast are:

• Whole wheat toast with sugar-free fruit spread

• Cantaloup (but not without eating something else)

• Whole Grain Cereals (check sugar levels)

• Non-fat, sugar-free yogurt

• Skim milk.

• Tomato Juice

Also consider non-breakfast items for breakfast. I have been known to eat leftover casseroles and other non-traditional foods for breakfast. The idea is to ensure that you consume some complex carbohydrates to give you energy during the day.

Lunch, dinner and snacks:

Burritos Galore!

I love burritos because they are versatile and can be made quickly. I have come up with several versions that are healthy, filling and guilt-free. These are also a fantastic way to use up leftovers.

Baked Chicken Burrito

Soft Tortilla Shells (Use corn or wheat and fat-free if you can get them)

Cut up chunks of baked chicken (I use leftovers)
Boiled Rice (brown rice is better)
Red kidney beans
Steamed broccoli, cut in small pieces
Fat-free cheddar *or* Mozzarella Cheese
Fat-free yogurt dressing* (recipe below)

Warm the tortilla shell to make it easier to roll. Spoon the baked chicken, rice, broccoli, kidney beans and cheese on the middle of the shell. Drizzle fat-free yogurt dressing over the other ingredients. Roll the burrito.

Vegetable Roll-Ups

Tortilla Shells
Shredded fresh spinach (lettuce can also be used)
Shredded Carrots
Bean Sprouts
Diced Tomatoes
Diced Bell Peppers
Non-fat Yogurt Dressing* (see below)

Warm the tortilla shells if they have been refrigerated to make them easier to roll. Pile on generous portions of the vegetables. Add your favorite non-fat or light dressing and enjoy! A great alternative to an ordinary salad.

Fat-free Yogurt Dressing

½ cup fat-free, unsweetened plain yogurt
½ cup chopped cucumber **or** celery
        (depending on your taste)
¼ cup chopped tomatoes
        (about 5 cherry tomatoes)
½ teaspoon dill weed
¼ teaspoon oregano
¼ teaspoon basil
pinch of freshly ground pepper

Toss all the ingredients into a blender and process until desired consistency. Using celery rather than the cucumber gives the dressing more texture. Feel free to add other veggies to make this dressing your own specialty.

Tomato and Cucumber Salad

Simple, yet delicious! Eat as much as you want.

Very finely sliced cucumbers, with skins intact
Chopped tomatoes
Light Italian dressing or yogurt dressing
Dill seed (to taste)

Toss the cucumber slices and tomatoes in a serving bowl. Sprinkle on a generous amount of dill seed. (A few teaspoons, depending on taste.) Add the dressing and toss. The dill seed brings out a wonderful flavor in the tomatoes and cucumbers. One of my favorite guilt-free foods!

Hearty Cold Pasta Salad

1 lb. pasta ("shaped" pastas like bow-tie work well), cooked and cooled
1 can of red kidney beans
1 cup chopped bell peppers
1 cup of chopped broccoli (steamed and cooled)
1 cup of cooked carrots (cooled and chopped)
Fat-free or light Italian dressing
2 tsp. Oregano
Pepper and Salt to taste

Prepare pasta according to directions. Cool by running cold water over the pasta. This will also prevent the pasta from continuing to cook. Add all other ingredients and toss. This is a colorful, appetizing salad that is hearty as well.

Desserts:

It is natural to have cravings for sweets. The problem for those of us with PCOS is that eating even a few sweets can have immediate negative results in the form of sluggishness, subsequent cravings, and additional weight gain.

Staying away from sugars, especially chocolate goodies has been my most challenging endeavor. Here are some of the foods that I indulge myself while keeping sugar and fat to a minimum.

- Fat-free, sugar-free instant puddings

- Sugar-free Jell-O
  (add fresh fruit before chilling and top with fat-free, sugar free whipped topping before serving)

- Frozen bananas on popsicle sticks

- Fruit Smoothies

(Smoothies are your own creation. Don't worry about exact measurements. Experiment with different fruits for a variety of textures and tastes.)

Note: Using frozen berries will makes your smoothies frosty without refrigerating or adding ice. Use fat-free plain yogurt to make a creamier smoothie.

Berry Cantaloupe Smoothie

½ cup diced cantaloupe
¼ cup blueberries
¼ cup strawberries
¼ cup raspberries

Toss all ingredients in a blender and process until desired consistency.

- Fresh Strawberries sprinkled with artificial sweetener or served with fat-free, sugar-free whipped topping.

- No-sugar added, fat-free ice creams and yogurt (always check the labels)

- No-sugar added applesauce sprinkled with cinnamon

- No-sugar added, fat-free cocoa (commercial packets)

Sometimes I like to "spike" my cocoa with an extra sprinkle of dry cocoa to make it taste even chocolatier. You could also top with a fat-free, no sugar added whipped topping.

Guilt-free Hot Cocoa

skim milk or water
1 tsp dry cocoa
2 tsp Splenda®
dash vanilla
dash salt

Mix dry ingredients in a mug. Add vanilla and either skim milk or water. Microwave for 2 minutes. When using water, this is virtually calorie free.

Additional recipes can be found:

- At your local library

- At your favorite bookstore

- On the Internet (see following chapter on web sites).

**It's not that I'm so smart,
it's just that I stay with problems longer.**

*Albert Einstein
1879-1955, German-born American Physicist*

Chapter 15
Additional Information

The following list contains resources for additional information.

Support Groups:

Polycystic Ovarian Syndrome Association

Rosemont IL   (630) 585-3690
60018-7007   www.pcosupport.org

Organizations:

American Diabetes Association

1-800-DIABETES (1-800-342-2383)

ATTN: Customer Service
1660 Duke Street
Alexandria, VA 22314

www.diabetes.org
customerservice@diabetes.org

American Heart Association

Customer Heart and Stroke Information:
1-800-AHA-USA1

Women's Health Information:
1-888-MY-HEART
www.women.americanheart.org

The American Society for Reproductive Medicine
(Formerly The American Fertility Society)

American Society for Reproductive Medicine
1209 Montgomery Highway   Birmingham, Alabama
35216-2809

asrm@asrm.org
www.asrm.org
(205) 978-5000
Fax: (205) 978-5005

Center for Applied Reproductive Science

Johnson City Medical Center Office Building   408 State
of Franklin Rd.
Johnson City, Tennessee   37604

Info@ivf-et.com
www.ivf-et.com

423-461-8880
Fax: 423-461-8887

The Endocrine Society

The Endocrine Society
4350 East West Highway,
Suite 500
Bethesda, MD 20814-4426

members@endo-society.org
www.endo-society.org
1-800-ENDO-SOC
(International: 1-301-941-0210)

Fax: 301-941-0259

The Journal of Reproductive Medicine

The Journal of Reproductive Medicine
P.O. Drawer 12425
8342 Olive Blvd.
St. Louis, MO 63132

(314) 991-4440
Fax: (314) 991-4654
editor@jreprodmed.com
reprints@jreprodmed.com
subscriptions@jreprodmed.com
www.jreprodmed.com/

Educational Web sites:

A Forum for Women's Health

Internet resource for women's health information.

www.womenshealth.org

The American Medical Women's Association

This site includes information about women in medicine and links to home pages of the American Medical Association and the Journal of the American Medical Association.

www.amwa-doc.org

Health Finder

This web site from the Department of Health and Human Services provides direct links to online publications and databases, including consumer health information from Federal agencies.

www.healthfinder.gov

Health Insight: Women's Health

General health information for women from the American Medical Association's Health Insight.

www.ama-assn.org/insight/h_focus/wom_hlth/wom_hlth.htm

JAMA Women's Health Information Center

The Women's Health Information Center maintained by the Journal of the American Medical Association. The site is designed as a resource for physicians and other health professionals but is open to the general public.

www.ama-assn.org/special/womh/womh.htm

Mayo Health O@sis Women's Health Resource Center

The Women's Health Resource Center of the Mayo Clinic's Health Oasis includes material like Mayo Clinic articles and offers colorful and detailed graphics and glossary.

www.mayo.ivi.com/mayo/common/htm/womenpg.htm

The New York Times on the Web - Women's Health

www.nytimes.com/specials/women/whome/index.html

Society for the Advancement of Women's Health Research

The web site for a non-profit organization founded in 1990 to campaign for more research on women's health.

www.womens-health.org

The Wellness Web's Women's Health Page

The Wellness Web's Women's Health Page is set up and monitored by patients and allows users to chat with other patients. It refers users to sources that range from the Journal of the American Medical Association to patient accounts (more carefully screened than those on Medweb) on issues like smoking during pregnancy and premenstrual syndrome. Visit the Wellness Web main site at www.wellweb.com for general health information.

www.wellweb.com/WOMEN/WOMEN.HTM

Women's Health: Information from your family doctor

Information on frequently asked questions from the American Academy of Family Physicians.

www.aafp.org/patientinfo/health4.html

Websites on Coronary Artery Disease:

Facts About Heart Disease and Women: Be Physically Active

A pamphlet from the National Heart, Lung and Blood Institute.

www.nhlbi.nih.gov/nhlbi/cardio/other/gp/hdw_act.htm

Intelihealth: Women and Heart Disease

Information from Johns Hopkins.

www.intelihealth.com/cgi-bin/returntofr.cgi?http://www.inteliheal th.com/specials/htWomen.htm?r=WSNYT000

Take Wellness to Heart

Information for women on heart disease and stroke, from the American Heart Association.

women.americanheart.org

Women's Cardiovascular Institute of Southern California

Information on women and cardiovascular disease from a Los Angeles-based prevention, diagnosis and treatment institute.

www.hygeia.com/institute

Websites on Nutrition, Fitness and General Health Issues:

Diet & Nutrition Resource Center

This Mayó Health O@sis resource center provides an index of reference articles, a "virtual cookbook" of healthy recipes, quizzes on nutritional information and links to other web sites.

www.mayo.ivi.com/mayo/common/htm/dietpage.htm

Health Insight: Fitness Basics

Information on fitness and exercise, from the American Medical Association's Health Insight.

www.ama-assn.org/insight/gen_hlth/fitness/fitness.htm

Health Insight: Interactive Health

Evaluate your eating habits, weight and fitness regimen with tools from the American Medical Association's Health Insight.

www.ama-assn.org/consumer/interact.htm

Nutrition and Obesity Publications Online

Pamphlets on topics such as binge eating, obesity drugs and very low calorie diets from the National Institute of Diabetes and Digestive and Kidney Diseases' Weight-control Information Network.

www.niddk.nih.gov/health/nutrit/nutrit.htm

Nutrition and Your Health: Dietary Guidelines for Americans

Guidelines from the U.S. Department of Health and Human Services and the U.S. Dept. of Agriculture

www.nalusda.gov/fnic/dga/dguide95.html

Physical Activity and Health: A Report of the Surgeon General

A 1996 report assessing research on the links between physical activity and health and offering guidelines for ways communities can encourage exercise.

www.cdc.gov/nccdphp/sgr/sgr.htm

Reproduction Issues:

Assisted Reproductive Technology Success Rates

Latest information from the Centers for Disease Control and Prevention.

www.cdc.gov/nccdphp/drh/arts

National Center for Human Reproduction

www.centerforhumanreprod.com

Endnotes

1)   Editors, "Polycystic Ovary Syndrome: The Story", <u>HealthNews</u> , July 25, 1998, p. 4.

2)   Ar, Dr. Bob, "Help Fighting Ovarian Cysts", NBC NE, Dec. 1998 story, www.msnbc.com/ news/221511.asp.

3,4)   "Polycystic Ovary Syndrome and You"; University of Pittsburgh; www.pitt.edu/ %7Ekerst9/pcopage.htm.

5)   Dunaif, Dr. Andrea, MD, "The Physician's Perspective", <u>HealthNews</u>, p. 4.

6)   Ar, Dr. Bob, "Help Fighting Ovarian Cysts", NBC NE, Dec. 1998 story, www.msnbc.com/ news/221511.asp.

7)   Dunaif, Dr. Andrea, MD, "The Physician's Perspective", <u>HealthNews</u>, p. 4.

8)   Kidson, Warren, "Polycystic Ovary Syndrome: A New Direction in Treatment", MJA 1998; 169: 537-540.

9,10)   Dunaif, Dr. Andrea, MD, "The Physician's Perspective", <u>HealthNews</u>, p. 4.

11)   "Defining PCOS", University of Chicago Center for Polycystic Ovary Syndrome; http://centerforpcos.bsd.uchicago.edu/Defining_PCOS/defining_pcos.html.

12,13)   "Polycystic Ovary Syndrome and You"; University of Pittsburgh; www.pitt.edu/ %7Ekerst9/pcopage.htm.

14)   Legro, Richard S.; Kunselman, Allen R.; Dodson, William C. ; and Dunaif, Andrea; "Prevalence and Predictors of Risk for Type 2 Diabetes Mellitus and Impaired Glucose Tolerance in Polycystic Ovary Syndrome: A Prospective, Controlled Study in 254 Affected Women"; <u>The Journal of Clinical Endocrinology & Metabolism</u>; January 1999; Volume 84, Number 1, Pages 165 - 169.

15)   Nestler, Dr. John E. , MD; "Fertility: An Insulin Resistance Problem?: Polycystic Ovary Syndrome: The Insulin Story";

Session Summary from 1-22-99; www.diabetes.org/pg99/ sessions/nestler.asp.

16)   "Defining PCOS", University of Chicago Center for Polycystic Ovary Syndrome; http://centerforpcos.bsd.uchicago.edu/Defining_PCOS/defi ning_pcos.html.

17-19)   "Polycystic Ovary Syndrome and You"; University of Pittsburgh; www.pitt.edu/ %7Ekerst9/pcopage.htm.

20-23)   "Tracing Ovarian Cysts Back to the Womb"; Doctor's Guide to Medical & Other News; London, England; 10-17-97.

24,25)   "Defining PCOS", University of Chicago Center for Polycystic Ovary Syndrome; http://centerforpcos.bsd.uchicago.edu/Defining_PCOS/defi ning_pcos.html.

26)   "Polycystic Ovary Syndrome and You"; University of Pittsburgh; www.pitt.edu /%7Ekerst9/pcopage.htm.

27-29)   Glueck, Charles J., MD, "Polycystic Ovary Syndrome"; The Cholesterol Center; blues.fd1.uc.edu/~gartsips/polycyst.htm.

30,31)   Ezrin, Dr. Calvin, MD; "Doctor to Doctor: Hyperinsulinism: The Metabolic Trap in Resistant Obesity"; includes references to Chapter 14 "The Type II Diabetes book", 1995, Lowell House Publishers CA; http://commodore.perry.pps.pgh.pa.us/~odonnell/ezrin.html.

32)   Discussion: Message Boards, Polycystic Ovarian Syndrome Association, www.pcosupport.org/.

33,34)   Ezrin, Dr. Calvin, MD; "Doctor to Doctor: Hyperinsulinism: The Metabolic Trap in Resistant Obesity"; includes references to Chapter 14 "The Type II Diabetes book", 1995, Lowell House Publishers CA; http://commodore.perry.pps.pgh.pa.us/~odonnell/ezrin.html.

35)   "Polycystic Ovary Syndrome and You"; University of Pittsburgh; www.pitt.edu/ %7Ekerst9/pcopage.htm.

36,37)   Ezrin, Dr. Calvin, MD; "Doctor to Doctor: Hyperinsulinism: The Metabolic Trap in Resistant Obesity"; includes references to Chapter 14 "The Type II Diabetes book", 1995, Lowell House Publishers CA; http://commodore.perry.pps.pgh.pa.us/~odonnell/ezrin.html.

38-40)   "What is Insulin Resistance"; IR-Web General Public Section; http://www.ir-web.com/ english/gp/ir/irmenu1/ irmenu1.asp.

41)   Kidson, Warren, "Polycystic Ovary Syndrome: A New Direction in Treatment", MJA 1998; 169: 537-540.

42)   Perloe, Dr. Mark, MD; "Polycystic Ovary Syndrome: Treatment with Insulin Lowering Medications"; Atlanta Reproductive Health Centre WWW; www.ivf.com/pcostreat.html.

43,45)   Calechman, Steve; "Age Proofing"; *Natual Health,* September 2000, p. 118.

44)   Nestler, Dr. John E. , MD; "Fertility: An Insulin Resistance Problem?: Polycystic Ovary Syndrome: The Insulin Story"; Session Summary from 1-22-99; www.diabetes.org/ pg99/sessions/ nestler.asp.

46)   Ezrin, Dr. Calvin, MD; "Doctor to Doctor: Hyperinsulinism: The Metabolic Trap in Resistant Obesity"; includes references to Chapter 14 "The Type II Diabetes book", 1995, Lowell House Publishers CA; http://commodore.perry.pps.pgh.pa.us/~odonnell/ezrin.html.

47)   Robbins, Anthony, "Personal Power", Audio Series.

48,49)   Kidson, Warren, "Polycystic Ovary Syndrome: A New Direction in Treatment", MJA 1998; 169: 537-540.

50)   Perloe, Dr. Mark, MD; "Polycystic Ovary Syndrome: Treatment with Insulin Lowering Medications"; Atlanta Reproductive Health Centre WWW; www.ivf.com/pcostreat.html.

51)   Nestler, Dr. John E. , MD; "Fertility: An Insulin Resistance Problem?: Polycystic Ovary Syndrome: The Insulin Story";

Session Summary from 1-22-99; www.diabetes.org/pg99/
sessions/nestler.asp.

52,53)   "New Insulin-Sensitizer Looks Promising"; News Stories;
          S o u r c e :   M e d i c a l   T r i b u n e ;
          www.diabetes.com/morenews/news_980909.htm.

54,55)   Perloe, Dr. Mark, MD; "Polycystic Ovary Syndrome:
          Treatment with Insulin Lowering Medications"; Atlanta
          R e p r o d u c t i v e   H e a l t h   C e n t r e   W W W ;
          www.ivf.com/pcostreat.html.

56,57)   Glueck, Charles J., MD, "Polycystic Ovary Syndrome"; The
          Cholesterol Center; blues.fd1.uc.edu/~gartsips/polycyst.htm.

58-60)   "Drug Effective in Treating Polycystic Ovary Syndrome";
          ADA   Conference;   Chicago,   June   15,   1998;
          www.pslgroup.com/dg/84f7e.htm.

61-63)   "New Insulin-Sensitizer Looks Promising"; News Stories;
          S o u r c e :   M e d i c a l   T r i b u n e ;
          www.diabetes.com/morenews/news_980909.htm.

64)   Ezrin, Dr. Calvin, MD; "Doctor to Doctor: Hyperinsulinism:
          The Metabolic Trap in Resistant Obesity"; includes references
          to Chapter 14 "The Type II Diabetes book", 1995, Lowell
          H o u s e   P u b l i s h e r s   C A ;
          http://commodore.perry.pps.pgh.pa.us/~odonnell/ezrin.html.

65)   Richwine, Lisa, "US panel says diabetes drug should stay on
          market"; Reuters, Bethesda, Md., March 26, 1999.

66-71)   Perloe, Dr. Mark, MD; "Polycystic Ovary Syndrome:
          Treatment with Insulin Lowering Medications"; Atlanta
          R e p r o d u c t i v e   H e a l t h   C e n t r e   W W W ;
          www.ivf.com/pcostreat.html.

Bibliography

"ADA Conference: Drug Effective in Treating Polycystic Ovary Syndrome"; Chicago, June 15, 1998; www.pslgroup.com/dg/84f7e.htm.

Ar, Dr. Bob. "Help Fighting Ovarian Cysts", NBC NE, Dec. 1998 story, www.msnbc.com/news/ 221511.asp.

Calechman, Steve. "Age Proofing", Natural Health, Sept. 2000, p.118.

"Defining PCOS", University of Chicago Center for Polycystic Ovary Syndrome; http://centerforpcos.bsd. uchicago.edu/Defining_PCOS/defining_pcos.html.

Discussion: Message Boards, Polycystic Ovarian Syndrome Association, http://www.pcosupport.org/.

Dunaif, MD, Dr. Andrea. "The Physician's Perspective", HealthNews, p. 4.

Editors. "Polycystic Ovary Syndrome: The Story", HealthNews , July 25, 1998, p. 4.

Ezrin, MD, Dr. Calvin. "Doctor to Doctor: Hyperinsulinism: The Metabolic Trap in Resistant Obesity"; includes references to Chapter 14 "The Type II Diabetes book", 1995, Lowell House Publishers CA; http://commodore.perry.pps.pgh.pa.us/~odonnell/ ezrin.html.

Glueck, MD, Charles J. "Polycystic Ovary Syndrome"; The Cholesterol Center; blues.fd1.uc.edu/~gartsips/ polycyst.htm.

Kidson, Warren. "Polycystic Ovary Syndrome: A New Direction in Treatment", MJA 1998; 169: 537-540.

Legro, Richard S.; Kunselman, Allen R.; Dodson, William C. ; and Dunaif, Andrea. "Prevalence and Predictors of Risk for Type 2 Diabetes Mellitus and Impaired Glucose Tolerance in Polycystic Ovary Syndrome: A Prospective, Controlled Study in 254 Affected Women";

The Journal of Clinical Endocrinology & Metabolism; January 1999; Volume 84, Number 1, Pages 165 - 169.

"New Insulin-Sensitizer Looks Promising"; News Stories; Source: Medical Tribune; www.diabetes.com/morenews/ news_980909.htm.

Nestler, MD. Dr. John E.   "Fertility: An Insulin Resistance Problem?: Polycystic Ovary Syndrome: The Insulin Story"; Session Summary from 1-22-99; www.diabetes.org/pg99/ sessions/nestler.asp.

Perloe, MD, Dr. Mark.   "Polycystic Ovary Syndrome: Treatment with Insulin Lowering Medications"; Atlanta Reproductive Health Centre WWW; www.ivf.com/ pcostreat.html.

"Polycystic Ovary Syndrome and You"; University of Pittsburgh; www.pitt.edu/%7Ekerst9/ pcopage.htm.

Richwine, Lisa. "US panel says diabetes drug should stay on market"; Bethesda, Md., March 26, 1999, Reuters.

Robbins, Anthony. "Personal Power", Audio Series.

"Tracing Ovarian Cysts Back to the Womb"; Doctor's Guide to Medical & Other News; London, England; 10-17-97.

Printed in the United States
16558LVS00005B/215